King's Applied Anatomy of the
Abdomen and Pelvis
of Domestic Mammals

# King's Applied Anatomy of the Abdomen and Pelvis of Domestic Mammals

*Geoff Skerritt, BVSc, FRSB, DipECVN, FRCVS*
*Royal College of Veterinary Surgeons*
*Specialist and European Specialist in*
*Veterinary Neurology*
*Chester, UK*


*With invited contribution from:*

*J. David Stack, MVB, MSc, FHEA, DipECVS, MRCVS*
*Senior Lecturer in Equine Surgery*
*University of Liverpool*
*Leahurst, UK*

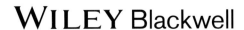

This edition first published 2022
© 2022 John Wiley & Sons Ltd

*Registered Offices*
John Wiley & Sons, Inc., 111 River Street, Hoboken, NJ 07030, USA
John Wiley & Sons Ltd, The Atrium, Southern Gate, Chichester, West Sussex, PO19 8SQ, UK

*Editorial Office*
9600 Garsington Road, Oxford, OX4 2DQ, UK

For details of our global editorial offices, customer services, and more information about Wiley products visit us at
www.wiley.com.

Wiley also publishes its books in a variety of electronic formats and by print-on-demand. Some content that appears in
standard print versions of this book may not be available in other formats.

*Library of Congress Cataloging-in-Publication Data*

Names: Skerritt, G. C. author.
Title: King's applied anatomy of the abdomen and pelvis of domestic mammals
    / Geoff Skerritt.
Other titles: Applied anatomy of the abdomen and pelvis of domestic mammals
Description: First edition. | Hoboken, NJ : John Wiley & Sons, 2022. |
    Includes bibliographical references and index.
Identifiers: LCCN 2021060395 (print) | LCCN 2021060396 (ebook) | ISBN
    9781119574576 (paperback) | ISBN 9781119574583 (adobe pdf) | ISBN
    9781119574590 (epub)
Subjects: MESH: Animals, Domestic–anatomy & histology | Abdomen–anatomy &
    histology | Pelvis–anatomy & histology
Classification: LCC SF761 (print) | LCC SF761  (ebook) | NLM SF 761 | DDC
    636.089/1–dc23/eng/20220119
LC record available at https://lccn.loc.gov/2021060395
LC ebook record available at https://lccn.loc.gov/2021060396

Cover design by: Wiley
Cover image: © Geoff Skerritt

Set in 10/12pt Warnock Pro by Straive, Pondicherry, India

Printed in Singapore
M096305_310122

*I wish to dedicate this book to the late Professor Tony King in recognition of his enthusiasm for the teaching of veterinary anatomy. It was his encouragement to teach anatomy in an original and inventive manner that gave me the incentive to make the subject interesting!*

# Contents

# Foreword

This publication is the latest of a series of textbooks the first of which was written by the late Professor A.S. King and colleagues. This series is now being continued by Geoff Skerritt. These textbooks and lecture notes initially were aimed at undergraduate veterinary students at the University of Liverpool. Professor King was always concerned to make anatomy useful by emphasising its functional importance so that students and veterinary professionals could acquire the basis for understanding the rationale of clinical practice in all its aspects.

This functional approach is continued by Geoff Skerritt, with emphasis on modern imaging techniques and is complemented by concise clearly illustrated anatomic details. The author of this new publication, and the writer of this foreword, as colleagues of Tony King, have experienced the benefit of this functional approach to anatomy. This approach is likely to be of continuing benefit to the present generation of students and veterinary professionals.

*Donald Kelly*
Emeritus Professor of Veterinary Pathology
University of Liverpool
Leahurst, UK

# Preface

The origin of this book is linked to the similar text on the *Applied Anatomy of the Central Nervous System* and to the earlier book on the *Functional Anatomy of the Limbs*. These books were based on the undergraduate courses on applied veterinary anatomy that were given to Liverpool University veterinary students from 1970 onwards. The Department of Veterinary Anatomy during this time was staffed by a group of enthusiastic staff members who were responsible for a highly successful undergraduate course given to first-year veterinary students. Professor Anthony King was the driving force that made veterinary anatomy a popular start to the careers in veterinary science. The success of the veterinary anatomy course was largely due to the way that anatomy, previously a rather boring subject comprising pure factual knowledge, became interesting and illustrated with applied and clinical facts that held the attention of the students. It was inevitable that the lecture notes that the staff produced to illustrate their lectures and practical classes should form the basis for more formal public interest and benefit from regular updating. Applied anatomy began to have a place in the clinical years of the veterinary degree course and supportive publications followed.

This book on the applied anatomy of the abdomen and pelvis originated from the lectures given by Tony King, Dr Keith Benson and myself. We were fortunate to be joined by Dr John Cox, a member of the clinical staff and an expert on mammalian reproduction. John made a valuable contribution to the chapters on pelvic anatomy, and I am grateful for his help and enthusiasm. The book contains a selection of diagrams to illustrate the text, and I am indebted to my wife, Dr Judith Skerritt, for her patience and skill in developing most of these. Finally, I needed help with the section on recent advances in diagnostic procedures particularly in equine patients. I am grateful to Dr Dave Stack for filling the gap. He is a clinician with particular experience of modern diagnostic techniques especially in regard to equine patients.

Geoff Skerritt

# Acknowledgements

I would like to thank my wife, Judith, for her constant support and for her input into the illustrations. Wife, Judith, a mathematician, gave invaluable help to the computerisation of many of the figures so that they would be correct. She has helped me with the anatomical illustrations. Her skilfull use of the computer brought invaluable results to many otherwise typical anatomical diagrams.

John Cox is retired but was a popular member of staff at the Liverpool Veterinary School, where he taught and researched reproduction of domestic animals. Tony King recognised John's enthusiasm for teaching the clinical application of applied anatomy in the early years of the veterinary course. I am grateful to John for his contribution and advice in the area of pelvic anatomy.

Dave Stack is a more recent member of staff at Liverpool. I am grateful to him for his knowledgable contribution in equine reproduction and especially for his provision of photographic illustrations.

## About the Author

**Dr Geoff Skerritt, BVSc, FRSB, DipECVN, FRCVS**
Dr Skerritt is a former lecturer in veterinary anatomy at the University of Liverpool and former principal at ChesterGates Veterinary Hospital, Chester. He was president of the British Veterinary Hospital Association from 2012 to 2014 and president of the European College of Veterinary Neurology from 1997 to 1990. He is a European Specialist in Veterinary Neurology, and he was a member of the Council of the Royal College of Veterinary Surgeons 1997–2010 and chairman of the Specialisation and Further Education Committee.

## About the Contributors

**Dr John Cox, BSc, BVetMed, PhD, FRCVS,** was formerly senior lecturer in veterinary science at the Universty of Liverpool, Leahurst. John provided the basis for chapters 15 and 16.

**Dr John David Stack, MVB, MSc, FHEA, DipECVS, MRCVS** is a senior lecturer in equine surgery at the University of Liverpool, Leahurst. David wrote the sections in chapter 18 on equine diagnostic imaging and laparoscopy.

**Dr Judith O.Skerritt, BSc, MSc, PhD., Childer Thornton, Cheshire.** She was formerly a partner and the business director of ChesterGates Veterinary Hospital.

## About the Companion Website

This book is accompanied by a companion website.

**www.wiley.com/go/skerritt/abdomen**

This website includes:

- Downloadable figure PowerPoint slides from the book.
- Multiple-choice questions to aid learning.

# 1

# The Boundaries of the Abdomen

## 1.1   Introduction

The abdomen is the major cavity of the body in the domestic animals and human beings. It contains the gastrointestinal tract, the liver, spleen, pancreas, kidneys and the ovaries together with most of the female reproductive tract. The abdomen is separated from the thorax cranially by the **diaphragm** and the caudal ribs; caudally it is continuous with the pelvic cavity.

Dorsally the abdomen is bounded by the **vertebrae**. Laterally and ventrally the boundaries of the abdomen comprise the **abdominal wall**, a soft tissue structure consisting of muscle, connective tissue and the layers of the skin. The abdominal wall is capable of stretching in the short term, as when the gastrointestinal tract is full of ingesta, and more gradually to accommodate the expanding uterus in pregnancy.

Apart from the important functions of containing and protecting the abdominal contents, the muscular components of the abdominal wall can aid in the expulsion of faeces, urine and foetuses. In addition, contraction of the abdominal muscles can assist in breathing, coughing and sneezing.

## 1.2   The Diaphragm (Figure 8.3)

The diaphragm is the musculotendinous structure that separates the thoracic and abdominal cavities. It is dome-shaped with its apex pointing cranially. In the dog the diaphragm attaches to the **sternum** cranial to the **xiphoid cartilage** and to the medial surface of the 8th–13th ribs in the dog and cat. NB the horse has 18 pairs of ribs, ruminants 13, pigs 13–16. Dorsally the diaphragm attaches via the left and right crura to the third and fourth lumbar vertebrae. Dorsally the aorta, azygos vein and thoracic duct pass between the crura at the aortic hiatus. The oesophagus and the vagus nerves pass through the oesophageal hiatus located towards the centre of the diaphragm. The caval foramen (portal vena cava) is located on the right side of the central tendinous part of the diaphragm. Herniation of the diaphragm can occur as the result of trauma (see Section 1.7.4).

*King's Applied Anatomy of the Abdomen and Pelvis of Domestic Mammals*, First Edition. Geoff Skerritt.
© 2022 John Wiley & Sons Ltd. Published 2022 by John Wiley & Sons Ltd.
Companion website: www.wiley.com/go/skerritt/abdomen

## 1.3 The Layers of the Abdominal Wall

Between the skin and the parietal peritoneum lie several layers of fascia and muscle. A proper appreciation of these layers, and the direction of their fibres, is important when making surgical incisions for entry to the abdominal cavity.

### 1.3.1 The skin

The skin, or common integument, varies in thickness between species and bodily location. The abdominal skin is very thick (4–5 mm) in the ox but is quite delicate and thin (1–3 mm) in the other domestic species. Hair grows from the skin in all of the species but is much less in the pig. In all species there is much less hair on the ventral abdomen than elsewhere. Most of the hair of the sheep has a specific structure and is termed wool. In all species except the pig a principal function of the hair/wool is to reduce heat loss; the pig relies on a large amount of subcutaneous fat for this function.

The domestic species vary in regard to the number and distribution of the mammary glands. The mare has only two mammary glands, and these are located either side of the midline on the ventral abdomen in a prepubic position. The cow usually has four mammary glands, collectively known as the udder; it is located mainly ventral to the caudal abdomen but with its caudal part ventral to the pelvis. The udder is suspended by strong elastic tissue extending essentially from the **linea alba** and the symphyseal tendon.

There are seven pairs of mammary glands in the sow, although only 8–10 are usually functional depending on litter size. In this species the mammary tissue extends in the body wall from the axilla to the level of the stifle.

The udder of small ruminants comprises two glands and is situated in the inguinal region. In the bitch there are usually five pairs of mammary glands; in the cat there are generally four pairs.

### 1.3.2 The subcutaneous fascia

**Superficial fascia:** In the pig this layer is adipose over most of its area and functions as an insulating layer promoting heat retention. However, in most other species this adipose tissue is not complete except in the inguinal region. In horses and cattle the **cutaneous muscle** is well developed in the superficial fascia layer and serves to twitch the skin to dislodge flies.

**Deep fascia:** In the horse and ox the deep fascia is developed as a thick sheet of fibroelastic tissue covering most of the external abdominal oblique muscle, the ribs and the tuber coxae. This is termed the **yellow elastic tunic** providing support for the abdominal contents and contributing to the suspensory apparatus of the udder in the cow.

### 1.3.3 The rectus abdominis muscle (Figures 1.1 and 1.2)

Origin: The ventral surfaces of the sternal ribs and sternum.

Insertion: The cranial border of the pubis with the **prepubic tendon**. The prepubic tendon is the tendon of insertion of the two rectus abdominis muscles, although most of its fibres extend between the iliopubic eminences.

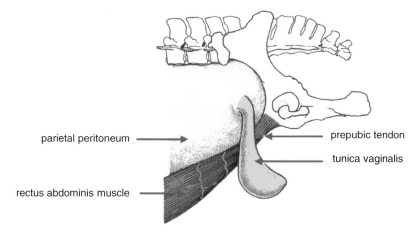

**Figure 1.1** Lateral view of inguinal region of horse showing the rectus abdominis muscle. The peritoneum of the vaginal tunic is strongly reinforced by fusion with the internal spermatic fascia (derived from the transverse abdominal muscle).

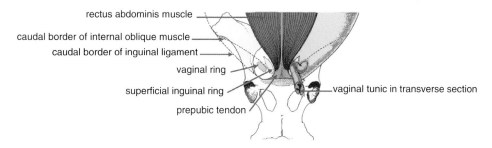

**Figure 1.2** Ventral view of the inguinal region of horse showing the rectus abdominis muscle. The left side of the diagram shows the relative positions of the superficial inguinal ring and the vaginal ring. On the right side of the diagram the vaginal tunic is shown wending its way from the deep inguinal ring, through the inguinal canal and out through the superficial inguinal ring.

Structure: The left and right muscles are separated longitudinally by the linea alba, a band of fibrous tissue extending from the xiphoid cartilage to the prepubic tendon. A series of three to six transverse tendinous inscriptions cross each muscle belly, but the resulting muscle segments are not correlated with the nerve supply.

**Species variations**: In the **ox** there is wide separation of the medial borders of the rectus abdominis muscles. caudally. In the immature animal the linea alba is perforated by the umbilicus.

## 1.3.4 External abdominal oblique muscle (Figures 1.3–1.5)

Origin: The lateral surfaces of the ribs caudal to the fourth rib and the lumbodorsal fascia.

Insertion: The linea alba and prepubic tendon.

Structure: Most of the muscle fibres run caudoventrally. At its origin it consists of muscle fibres but towards its insertion caudoventrally it becomes a tendinous

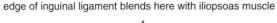

edge of inguinal ligament blends here with iliopsoas muscle

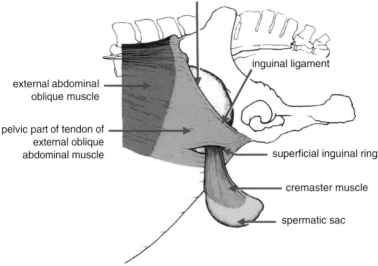

**Figure 1.3** Lateral view of the inguinal region of the horse left external oblique abdominal muscle. The spermatic sac is seen emerging from the left superficial inguinal ring. The spermatic sac contains the testicle and the spermatic cord (See Figure 15.4). For a definition of the spermatic sac see Section 16.4

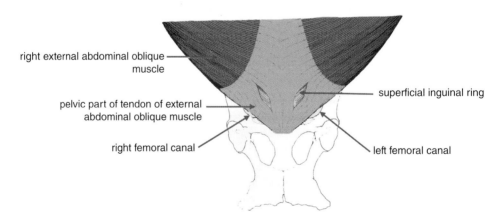

**Figure 1.4** Ventral view of inguinal region of the horse showing the left and right external abdominal oblique muscles. The arrows indicate the left and right femoral canals, providing exit for the femoral arteries and veins.

aponeurosis. Towards its insertion in the prepubic tendon there is a slit in the aponeurosis; this is the **superficial inguinal ring**. The slit divides the tendon into an abdominal part cranially and a pelvic part caudally. The caudal edge of the pelvic part of the tendon is the **inguinal ligament**.

**Species variations:** The external abdominal oblique muscle of the **dog** and **pig** is mainly muscular almost to the dorsal edge of the rectus abdominis muscle. In

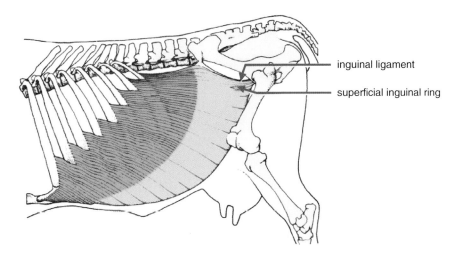

inguinal ligament

superficial inguinal ring

Figure 1.5  Lateral view of the abdomen of the ox showing the left external abdominal oblique muscle.

**ruminants** there is no origin from the lumbodorsal fascia, but there is an insertion on the tuber coxae. In the ox the aponeurosis of this muscle is extensive. In the **horse** the external abdominal oblique muscle is very large and inserts onto the femoral fascia, linea alba, tuber coxae and the prepubic tendon.

### 1.3.5   Internal abdominal oblique muscle (Figures 1.6–1.8)

Origin: Tuber coxae and lumbodorsal fascia.

Insertion: Linea alba (except for the most caudal part), last rib and cartilages of the caudal ribs.

Structure: This is a sheet of muscle and tendon with the fibres running cranioven-trally. It is muscular at its origin and becomes tendinous ventrally. In the male a slip of the internal abdominal oblique muscle passes through the inguinal canal on the lateral aspect of the vaginal process and becomes the cremaster muscle (see Section 16.4).

**Species variations**: The fibres of this muscle run almost ventrally in the **dog**. In carnivores the tendinous portion divides to pass dorsally and ventrally to the rectus abdominis muscle in the cranial third of the abdomen; it passes only ventrally in the caudal two-thirds of the abdomen. In the **ox** the internal abdominal oblique is quite substantial, being the largest flank muscle in this species; its tendon passes both ven-trally and dorsally to the rectus abdominis. In the **horse** the internal abdominal oblique muscle originates only from the tuber coxae, and its tendon passes ventrally to the rectus abdominis. See Figures 1.10a–c for a summary of the species variation of the sheath of the rectus abdominis.

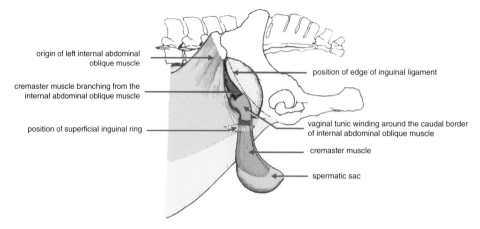

origin of left internal abdominal oblique muscle

cremaster muscle branching from the internal abdominal oblique muscle

position of superficial inguinal ring

position of edge of inguinal ligament

vaginal tunic winding around the caudal border of internal abdominal oblique muscle

cremaster muscle

spermatic sac

Figure 1.6 Lateral view of inguinal area of horse showing the internal abdominal oblique muscle. The left external abdominal oblique muscle has been removed although the position of the left superficial inguinal ring is shown. The mid-section of the left cremaster muscle has been excised to expose the vaginal tunic.

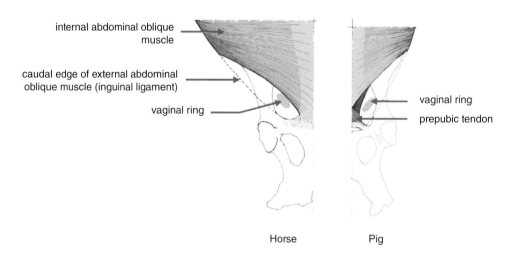

internal abdominal oblique muscle

caudal edge of external abdominal oblique muscle (inguinal ligament)

vaginal ring

vaginal ring

prepubic tendon

Horse          Pig

Figure 1.7 Ventral view of inguinal region showing internal abdominal oblique muscle.

### 1.3.6   Transverse abdominal muscle (Figure 1.9)

Origin: The medial surfaces of the ventral parts of the caudal ribs and the deep layers of the lumbodorsal fascia.

Insertion: The linea alba.

Structure: Again this muscle is sheet-like, although its fibres run ventrally and transversely to the longitudinal axis. Caudally the muscle thins out to only a fascial layer.

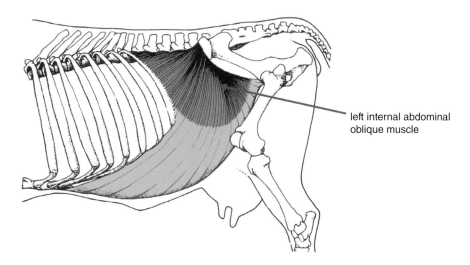

left internal abdominal
oblique muscle

Figure 1.8 Lateral view of abdomen of ox showing left abdominal oblique muscle. The external abdominal oblique has been removed.

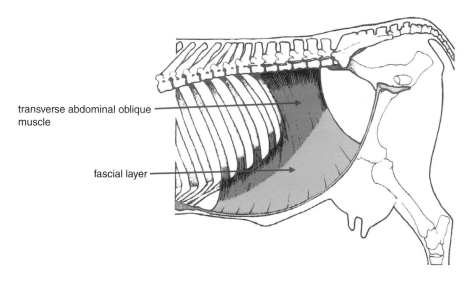

transverse abdominal oblique
muscle

fascial layer

Figure 1.9 Medial view of abdomen of ox showing the transverse abdominal muscle.

**Species variations:** In the **dog** the cranial two-thirds of the tendon pass dorsally to the rectus abdominis with the caudal third passing ventrally.

### 1.3.7 Retroperitoneal fascia

This tissue layer is equivalent to the superficial fascia but less defined. Its significance is due to its large fat content in the adult pig, fat ponies and beef breeds of cattle. Where the fascia is minimal the peritoneum is closely applied to the transverse abdominal muscle. The **falciform** ligament (see Sections 3.3 and 3.4) is a fold of peritoneum attached to the liver. It is a remnant of the peritoneum that contained the umbilical vein of the foetus; it attaches to the abdominal wall at the umbilicus.

### 1.3.8 Parietal peritoneum

This peritoneal layer lines the whole abdominal wall. It is a largely transparent and delicate layer that is reflected as mesenteries that are continuous with the visceral peritoneum that covers the abdominal viscera. The peritoneum comprises an outer layer of simple squamous epithelium called the mesothelium and is supported by a layer of loose connective tissue.

## 1.4 The Sheath of the Rectus Abdominis Muscle (Figures 1.10a–c)

The aponeuroses of the external, internal and transverse abdominal oblique muscles together form a sheath that encloses the rectus abdominis muscle either side of the midline of the abdominal wall. There are species differences and, in the dog, variations in the craniocaudal location.

**Species variations:** In the caudal third of the abdomen of the **dog** the tendon of the transverse abdominal muscle lies ventral to the rectus abdominis muscle. In the middle third of the abdomen the transverse abdominal tendon lies dorsal, and that of the internal abdominal oblique muscle passes ventral to the rectus abdominis (as in the **horse**). In the cranial third of the abdomen the tendon of the transverse abdominal muscle lies dorsal to the rectus muscle. In addition, the internal oblique tendon divides into a ventral and dorsal portion (as in the **ox**).

In the **horse** the aponeurosis of the internal oblique muscle lies ventral to the rectus abdominis. In addition, in this species, the yellow abdominal tunic is present.

In the **ox** the aponeurosis of the internal oblique divides to pass on both sides of the rectus abdominis, and a yellow abdominal tunic is again present. In this species the linea alba is particularly wide.

## 1.5 Clinical Importance of the Ventral Body Wall

A surgical incision in the abdominal wall is called a laparotomy. It may be made in the midline, to either side of the midline or in the flank on either side. The choice of location of the laparotomy depends on a number of factors:

i) The avascularity of the linea alba resulting in slow healing; this is a particular problem especially in cattle where the linea alba is extensive.
ii) The bulk and weight of the abdominal contents leading to slow healing and risk of herniation.
iii) In the dog the ventral sheath of the rectus abdominis is particularly strong, and failure to suture this may result in breakdown of a midline incision.
iv) In a midline incision contraction of the muscles of the abdominal wall tends to retract the wound edges laterally.

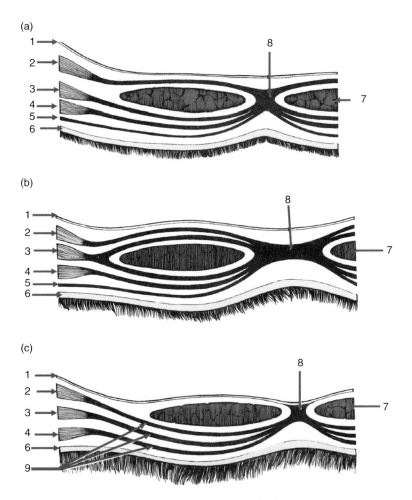

**Figure 1.10** Transverse sections through the ventral body wall to show the species variation in the sheath of the rectus abdominis. (a) The horse, (b) the ox and (c) the dog (caudal third of abdomen only). 1 = parietal peritoneum; 2 = transverse abdominis muscle; 3 = interior oblique abdominis muscle; 4 = exterior oblique abdominis muscle; 5 = yellow abdominis tunic; 6 = skin; 7 = rectus abdominis muscle; 8 = linea alba; 9 = ventral sheath of rectus abdominis muscle

v) Flank incisions should be parallel to the muscle fibres to minimise bleeding from the vascular muscular tissue.
vi) In the cow a further complication of a midline incision is that branches of the mammary vein may cross the midline to anastomose with the opposite mammary vein.

## 1.6   The Inguinal Canal (Figures 1.11 and 1.12)

The inguinal canal is a potential space extending between the superficial and deep inguinal rings. The canal does not have a surrounding wall. The external opening (superficial inguinal ring) is a slit in the aponeurosis thereby dividing it into two parts, an abdominal part (cranially) and a pelvic part (caudally).

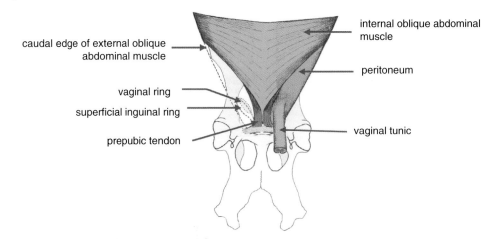

caudal edge of external oblique
abdominal muscle

internal oblique abdominal
muscle

peritoneum

vaginal ring

superficial inguinal ring

prepubic tendon

vaginal tunic

**Figure 1.11** Ventral view of inguinal canal of the pig. The left side of the diagram shows the superimposition of the superficial inguinal ring almost directly upon the vaginal ring in this species.

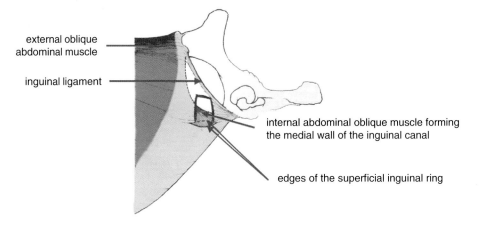

external oblique
abdominal muscle

inguinal ligament

internal abdominal oblique muscle forming
the medial wall of the inguinal canal

edges of the superficial inguinal ring

**Figure 1.12** Lateral view of the inguinal canal of the horse. A window has been cut from the pelvic part of the tendon of the external abdominal oblique muscle immediately adjoining the superficial inguinal ring. This exposes that part of the internal oblique abdominal muscle which forms the medial (deep) wall of the inguinal canal.

**Species variations**: The deep inguinal ring is different in the **pig** from that in the horse due to the different extent to which the internal oblique abdominal muscle inserts caudally. In the **horse** the deep inguinal ring is small, being bordered caudally by the inguinal ligament and cranially by the caudal edge of the internal oblique muscle (Figure 1.12) In the **pig** the deep inguinal ring is larger, bordered caudally by the inguinal ligament, cranially by the caudal edge of the internal abdominal oblique muscle and medially by the lateral border of the rectus abdominal muscle and the prepubic tendon (Figure 1.11). In the other domestic animals, the anatomy of the inguinal ring is between the horse and the pig but tends to be closer to the latter.

In the male foetus of all species an outpouching of parietal peritoneum, the **vaginal process** (Figure 16.6), enters the inguinal canal. The **gubernaculum** (see Section 16.9) develops from mesenchyme partly within the inguinal canal and joins the testes to the scrotum. In the adult male the inguinal canal contains the vaginal tunic, the cremaster muscle and the spermatic cord in addition to the external pudendal artery and vein, the inguinal lymph vessels and nerves. In the adult female it is only in the bitch that a rudimentary vaginal process extends through the inguinal canal.

## 1.7  Hernias

A hernia occurs when an organ or mesentery pushes through an opening in the muscle or tissue that normally holds it in place. Hernias occur most commonly in the abdomen when there is a deficit or weakness in the abdominal wall, but they may also occur at the diaphragm or the perineum. The several sites where hernias may occur are as follows:

1) Inguinal
2) Umbilical
3) Perineal
4) Diaphragmatic
5) Post-operative.

### 1.7.1  Inguinal hernia

The vaginal process develops in the embryo as an extension of the parietal peritoneum. Therefore the cavity of the vaginal process is continuous with the peritoneal cavity via the vaginal ring. In the male of all species and the bitch it is possible for abdominal contents (e.g. small intestine or great omentum) to protrude through the vaginal ring and enter the vaginal process. Within the vaginal process the herniated organ or tissue passes through the inguinal canal and may enter the scrotum. An inguinal hernia may or may not be reducible; an irreducible hernia may become strangulated if the blood supply becomes interrupted.

Congenital inguinal hernias are common in pigs, but in sheep they are thought to be a result of trauma. In the horse inheritance has not been proven, but they are more common in certain breeds.

### 1.7.2  Umbilical hernia

Normally, at birth, the umbilical ring closes and the umbilical blood vessels, the vitelline duct and the allantoic stalk begin to degenerate. If contraction of the umbilical ring does not occur completely it is possible for abdominal contents to enter the aperture and appear as a soft swelling beneath the umbilical scar.

### 1.7.3  Perineal hernia

The perineum is the part of the body wall that occludes the caudal opening of the pelvic cavity; it surrounds the anus and the urogenital opening. The major portion of the perineum, comprising the levator ani and coccygeus muscles, is called the **pelvic dia-phragm**. A hernia through the pelvic diaphragm can occur as a result of a defect in the musculature. This is a fairly complex anatomical area including the external anal sphincter, superficial gluteal muscle and sacrotuberous ligament.

Perineal hernias occur mainly in older male dogs and certain breeds, e.g. the Boxer, Boston Terrier, Pekingese and crossbreds.

### 1.7.4  Diaphragmatic hernia

The diaphragm separates the abdominal cavity from the thorax. Sudden increases in pressure in the abdomen can result in tears of the diaphragm with the consequence that abdominal organs can be forced into the thoracic cavity. This situation can occur as the result of a road traffic accident. Congenital hernias of the diaphragm are of rare occurrence in the dog and horse.

### 1.7.5  Post-operative hernia

A surgical incision in the abdominal wall is normally closed either with sutures or staples. If there is breakdown along the incision, there is a risk of herniation of abdominal organs. This situation may result from a variety of circumstances, e.g. poor healing of the incision due to inadequate vascularisation, pressure from the weight of the abdominal organs, faulty suturing technique and interference with the wound by the patient.

# 2

# Gastrointestinal Function

## 2.1 Introduction

In simple life forms, e.g. unicellular organisms such as the amoeba, food particles are ingested by a process of active envelopment with the resulting formation of a food vacuole within the cytoplasm. In higher orders of animal life this process plays no significant part in the process of digestion, although it is retained by **macrophage** cells in certain cellular activities such as **phagocytosis**, the ingestion or engulfing of particulate matter. Macrophages are a type of white blood cell found mainly in connective tissue and blood.

The development of the digestive tract involves cell specialisation occurring within the different regions of the tract and in relation to the functions of these different regions. Thus, while certain cells are specialised for absorbing food in a suitably processed form, other cells are primarily protective in function or are associated with transportation and with pre- treatment of the food to allow its utilisation. Further specialisation has evolved in relation to the nature of the food, so that marked variations occur in the gastrointestinal anatomy in herbivores as compared to carnivores. In general, however, the tract of higher vertebrates is divided into distinct anatomical regions, namely the buccal cavity, oesophagus, stomach, small intestines, large intestines and rectum. Further subdivisions of these regions are present.

## 2.2 Functions of the Alimentary Tract

These may be considered under the following four principal headings:

1) Transport
2) Physical treatment
3) Chemical treatment
4) Absorption.

### 2.2.1 Transport of food

Food transport, i.e. the active passage through the digestive tract, is promoted by the musculature that is located throughout the entire length of the digestive tract. There are two muscular coats comprising an inner circular and an outer longitudinal layer,

*King's Applied Anatomy of the Abdomen and Pelvis of Domestic Mammals*, First Edition. Geoff Skerritt.
© 2022 John Wiley & Sons Ltd. Published 2022 by John Wiley & Sons Ltd.
Companion website: www.wiley.com/go/skerritt/abdomen

together with a variable layer of oblique fibres. Contractions of the muscle layers promote the propulsion of food through the gastrointestinal tract, and segmental contractions ensure mixing of the intestinal contents.

In the oesophagus these layers are made up either wholly of striated skeletal muscle or partly of striated skeletal muscle and partly of smooth muscle. In the remainder of the tract the muscle layers comprise only smooth muscle innervated by the autonomic nervous system, which may either stimulate or inhibit muscular contraction. The muscle fibres can also operate independently of the nervous system; intermittent excitation is an intrinsic property of smooth muscle cells themselves, electrical transmission from muscle cell to muscle cell taking place at sites of low electrical resistance where one cell is in close apposition to another as at **gap junctions**. These are intimate connections between the cytoplasm of cells that allow the interchange of molecules, ions and electrical impulses.

Entry of food through the cardia into the stomach can occur following receptive relaxation of the smooth muscle of the gastric wall. The arrival of food **boluses,** round masses of food mixed with saliva, results in a vagal reflex that induces inhibition of muscle tone.

Transport is brought about by progressive waves of muscular contraction known as **peristalsis**. This results in a travelling constriction of the circular muscles arising at a point just cranial to the side of the food mass or **bolus** that has the effect of pushing the food caudally along the tract. Peristalsis occurs in the oesophagus, stomach and small intestines. Peristalsis also occurs in the large intestines, though the time interval between contractions is longer. An additional factor in the transport of food is the production of **mucus** by cells of the lining epithelium, thereby lubricating the passage of food along the intestines.

### 2.2.2  Physical treatment of food

To facilitate the action of enzymes upon the food taken into the digestive tract, it is necessary that the food be reduced to a soft pulp known as **chyme**. This is achieved largely by two types of contractile movement of the small intestines: (i) segmenting movements, which are single non-travelling constrictions of the muscular wall and have the effect of churning and mixing the food; and (ii) pendular movements that involve primary contractions of the longitudinal muscle and that induce marked shortening of individual loops of the intestines and consequently shaking the contained chyme from one end of the loop to another.

### 2.2.3  Chemical treatment of food

Water, salts and vitamins can be absorbed directly by the appropriate lining cells of the intestines, whereas enzymes and certain other substances are needed for the prior breakdown of proteins, carbohydrates and fats. These enzymes are produced and secreted by cells within the digestive tract, that is, by cells lining the stomach and intestines, and by glands external to the digestive tract. The latter comprise the salivary glands, liver and pancreas, which are derived embryologically from the developing digestive tract and are important sources not only of enzymes but also of other substances such as bile salts that are involved in the emulsification of fats. The production of enzymes to facilitate the breakdown of food in the digestive tract represents a marked degree of specialisation on the part of the cells concerned, since the enzymes are produced in large quantities and are then secreted to act beyond the confines of the producer cells. All body cells produce a variety of enzymes, but in general these act intracellularly.

An important additional facility to the above general mammalian pattern occurs in herbivores, where special provision is made for the breakdown of cellulose by bacterial fermentation, and in these species one portion of the digestive tract has structural modifications for this purpose; these modifications include the additional compartments of the stomach of the ruminant and the greatly enlarged caecum and colon of the horse.

### 2.2.4 Absorption

Following the physical and chemical treatment of the food and the breakdown of the major constituents into simple sugars, amino acids, fatty acids, etc., these relatively simple substances are absorbed by the columnar cells that line the small intestines and, to a lesser extent, the large intestines.

To facilitate absorption, and to increase the available surface area for absorption, various adaptations characterise the small intestines. The following are of particular significance: (i) in most mammalian species the small intestine is extremely long, as much as many times the length of the body. To accommodate this within the abdominal cavity, the small intestine is extensively coiled and is suspended as **festoons** by the peritoneal sheets of the mesentery. (ii) Crescentic folds of the internal lining membrane (the mucous membrane) occur, known as the **plicae circulares** (or the valves of Kerkring). (iii) Tiny finger-like projections of the lining mucous membrane are present in vast numbers along the length of the small intestine. They are covered by absorptive and mucus-secreting cells, and with a core of connective tissue, smooth muscle cells, blood vessels and **lacteals**, channels for transport of fat. These minute projections, known as villi, enormously increase the area for absorption. (iv) Finally, at the cellular level, at the luminal surface of each absorptive cell, the cell membrane is itself thrown into submicroscopic projections known as microvilli, which further increase the available absorptive surface.

## 2.3 Regions of the Alimentary Tract (Figure 2.1)

In the higher vertebrates the regions of the tract comprise the oesophagus, stomach, small intestine, large intestine and rectum. In ruminant herbivores (e.g. the ox) the stomach is very large and divided into four distinct regions, each with its own structure and function (see Sections 4.1 and 4.2.). The small intestine comprises the duodenum, jejunum and ileum (although these two divisions are ill-defined and are termed the jejunoileum). The large intestine in most species comprises a fairly long portion known as the colon, with a relatively short blind-ending diverticulum known as the caecum. However, there are wide species variations, and in some herbivores (e.g. the horse), the caecum is very large (see Section 6.2.1).

In lower vertebrates marked variations from the above pattern occur. For example, in several varieties of fish no stomach is present, there being only a single tube between

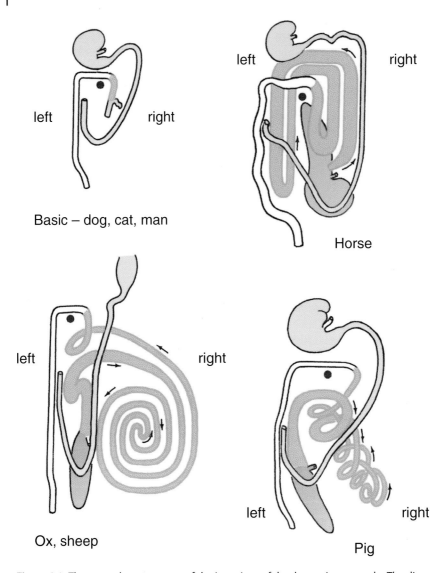

**Figure 2.1** The general arrangement of the intestines of the domestic mammals. The diagrams of the mammalian gastrointestinal tracts are drawn from the dorsal view although the ruminant intestinal spiral and the abomasum are displaced to the right by the rumen. The duodenum is V-shaped with the ascending limb lying dorsally on the right at the level of the base of the caecum (mauve). The stomach and the duodenum are both coloured green on the diagram. The jejunoileum is not shown on the diagram but occupies a large space between the duodenum and the colon mainly on the right. The transverse and descending colon retain their basic position. The transverse colon passes cranial to the root of the mesentery which contains the cranial mesenteric artery (red circle).

the pharynx and the intestine, which may be regarded as equivalent to the oesophagus. In fact the oesophagus only becomes well defined structurally in land vertebrates with the development away from gill breathing, i.e. an adaptation for the extraction of oxygen from water.

Important variations occur also in connection with the modifications to increase surface area mentioned earlier. Of particular importance, in view of its obvious functional success, is the so-called spiral intestine that characterises elasmobranch fishes. In these species the intestine is cigar-shaped and has a fold of internal epithelium projecting into the lumen. This projection twists spirally along the length of the intestine, thereby increasing the internal surface area. However, it seems that this adaptation is less successful than the greatly elongated intestine that is found in higher forms, from the teleost fishes to land vertebrates.

One feature that is common to the digestive tract of all vertebrates is the presence of a constriction known as the **pylorus**, which in most species occurs at the distal end of the stomach where the latter is continuous with the small intestine. The pylorus is a point of demarcation; that part of the tract cranial to the pylorus is known as the foregut and the region caudal to it is the hindgut. Primitively therefore the foregut was merely a short link between the pharynx and the intestine, with the latter being solely responsible for chemical treatment and absorption, but in higher orders the stomach has taken on an important role in this connection. It has developed as a storage area and for both the physical and chemical treatment of food. It seems likely that the development of this organ in an evolutionary sense is related to changed feeding habits, developing from primitive food strainers.

## 2.4   Clinical Conditions Affecting Gastrointestinal Function

The clinical presentation of gastrointestinal disease involves one or more of the following clinical signs (see Sections 4.3, 5.3, and 6.3):

1) Acute diarrhoea
2) Chronic diarrhoea
3) Vomiting
4) Weight loss
5) Abdominal discomfort
6) Anorexia
7) Presence of fresh or altered blood in the faeces.

Acute diarrhoea may be mild with no other clinical signs and due to a dietary trigger. Severe diarrhoea may result in dehydration, abdominal pain and a body temperature increase, and it may be due to an infection. Chronic diarrhoea, lasting more than 2 weeks, can have a variety of aetiologies ranging from neoplasia to hyperthyroidism (feline). Clinical signs such as increased or decreased frequency of defaecation or the presence of blood in the faeces are all diagnostically significant and may help in the localisation of intestinal disease.

A vomiting centre, located in the medulla oblongata of the hindbrain, mediates the vomiting reflex. The differential diagnosis of vomiting can be quite involved, although more so in dogs and cats rather than in the larger animals. Vomiting can be acute or chronic and may originate in the stomach or the small intestine; the possible causes are many and serious or trivial. Retching is followed by abdominal contractions resulting in forceful expulsion of oesophageal and gastric contents.

There are many possible causes of weight loss in animals. In dogs and cats disorders of malabsorption (see Section 5.3.5) may result from inflammatory bowel disease or severe parasitism. In farm animals there are a number of specific diseases that may cause weight loss, e.g. Johne's disease in cattle and sheep (see Sections 5.3.2 and 5.3.3).

Abdominal discomfort in animals is usually detected by the patient's restlessness and pain on palpation. In dogs gastroenteritis and gastric dilatation and volvulus (GDV) are severe causes of abdominal pain requiring urgent attention (see Section 4.3.5). In horses colic is a serious cause of abdominal pain (see Section 6.3).

Loss of appetite (anorexia) may have many causes in dogs ranging from dietary preference to a variety of causes warranting clinical assessment. In horses the explanation for a loss of appetite may be dental pain.

Haemorrhagic gastroenteritis is potentially a serious cause of blood in the faeces of dogs. Other possible causes are parasitism, parvovirus infection, *E. coli* infection and neoplasia.

# 3

# The Mesenteries, Ligaments and Omenta

The simple squamous epithelium that lines the abdominal and pelvic cavities is called the mesothelium; it is derived embryologically from the mesoderm. The outermost mesothelium, lining the internal surface of the body wall, is the **parietal peritoneum**. The innermost mesothelium, lining the outer surface of most of the abdominal and pelvic organs, is the **visceral peritoneum**. The two layers of peritoneum are continuous with one another at the **root of the mesentery**, which provides a short attachment to the abdominal wall. The cavity between the two layers of peritoneum is the **peritoneal cavity**. In the dog the root of the mesentery attaches to the body wall at the level of the second lumbar vertebra. With a few exceptions (e.g. kidneys and ovaries) each abdominal and pelvic organ is linked to the root of the mesentery by folds of mesentery called the mesojejunum, mesocolon, mesorectum, etc. The **great mesentery** is the collective term for the mesojejunum and mesoileum.

## 3.1 The Greater Omentum (Figure 3.1)

The **dorsal mesogastrium** attaches to the greater curvature of the stomach and grows caudally as a net-like cover over the ventral aspect of the intestines; it becomes the **greater omentum**. The greater omentum actually comprises two layers like a pouch with a parietal or superficial part and a visceral or deep part. The two layers extend cranially to the transverse colon, where they pass either side and form attachments to the pancreas and the spleen. The enclosed cavity is the **omental bursa** and has only one entry, the **epiploic foramen**, located caudomedial to the caudate lobe of the liver. The epiploic foramen is dorsal to the caudal vena cava and dorsomedial to the hepatic portal vein. It is slit-like and measures about 4 cm in the dog.

In the ruminants the deep layer of the greater omentum attaches just ventral to the right groove of the rumen. The superficial layer attaches to the left groove of the rumen so that the ventral sac lies within the omental bursa. The **supraomental recess** is the space dorsal to the deep layer of the great omentum in ruminants; it contains the intestines and opens caudally.

*King's Applied Anatomy of the Abdomen and Pelvis of Domestic Mammals*, First Edition. Geoff Skerritt.
© 2022 John Wiley & Sons Ltd. Published 2022 by John Wiley & Sons Ltd.
Companion website: www.wiley.com/go/skerritt/abdomen

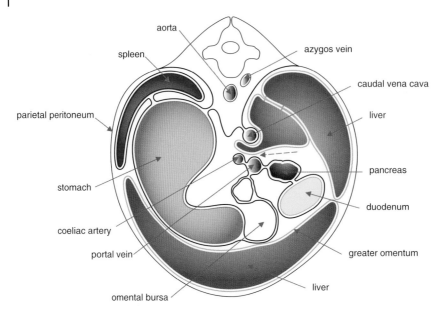

Figure 3.1 Transverse diagram of the abdomen to show the greater omentum, omental bursa and epiploic foramen (dashed arrow).

## 3.2 The Clinical Significance of the Greater Omentum

The greater omentum has several important functions:

1) It includes a network of blood vessels and lymphatic vessels that enable a rapid response to tackle foci of infection and inflammation. This function led the surgeon Rutherford Morison (1853–1939) to call the greater omentum the 'policeman of the abdomen'. Areas of infection can be isolated and further spread prevented.
2) Varying quantities of fat can be deposited. In man this can be excessive.
3) The greater omentum is a convenient insulating layer serving to avoid heat loss from the intestines.
4) The greater omentum can be wrapped around wounds surgically as a protective 'bandage'.

## 3.3 The Lesser Omentum

The **lesser omentum** and the **falciform ligament** are both developed from the ventral mesogastrium. The lesser omentum is the short stalk of ventral mesogastrium connecting the lesser curvature of the stomach to the visceral surface of the liver.

## 3.4 Ligaments

Mesenteries and omenta are folds of peritoneum. In addition, narrow strips of peritoneum are referred to as **ligaments**. They differ from ligaments associated with the skeleton in that they do not have attachments to bone. Examples are the gastrosplenic, hepatoduodenal, falciform, inguinal and ovarian ligaments. The attachments of these ligaments are usually indicated by their names.

### 3.4.1 Abdominal ligaments

The falciform ligament attaches to the parietal surface of the liver between the right and left medial lobes. Caudally it attaches to the body wall just cranial to the umbilicus. In young puppies a remnant of the umbilical vein, the teres ligament, is seen on the dorsal border of the falciform ligament. In the dog the falciform ligament becomes packed with fat and is often removed surgically to allow better access to the cranial abdomen.

The **round ligament of the liver** is a remnant of the umbilical vein of the foetus. It is only present in the young animal when it is there as a fibrous cord lying along the free edge of the falciform ligament.

The **coronary ligament** is present only as a peritoneal reflection between the liver and the caudal vena cava where it passes through the diaphragm.

The **hepatorenal ligament** extends from the caudate process of the liver to the ventral surface of the right kidney.

### 3.4.2 Pelvic ligaments

The **urachus** is a vestigial scar on the apex of the wall of the urinary bladder; it is the remains of the allantoic stalk that drains the nitrogenous waste from the embryonic urinary bladder to the placenta for excretion. The peritoneal fold that encloses the urachus becomes the **middle ligament** of the bladder. There are also, to either side, peritoneal folds that supported the umbilical arteries of the embryo; these become the **lateral ligaments** of the bladder. The umbilical arteries themselves become the **round ligaments** of the urinary bladder.

Blind-ending peritoneal pouches lie between the pelvic viscera and are directed caudally. They are named according to their attachments, which are also their boundaries. The **pubovesical pouch** (not usually present in the female) lies between the pelvis and the urinary bladder; the **rectogenital pouch** lies between the rectum and the reproductive tract; and the **vesicogenital pouch** lies between the bladder and the reproductive tract.

The gubernacula are paired embryonic ligaments derived from mesenchyme and also called the caudal genital ligaments. They are present in both the male and the female but have more functional significance in the male. In the female they become the ovarian and the round ligaments.

### 3.4.3 Pelvic ligaments – female

A number of ligaments are attached to the pelvic viscera. In the female these structures attach the female reproductive tract to the body wall. They are:

1) **Broad ligaments:** These are paired sheet-like double folds of peritoneum. They are attached dorsally to the body wall at the level of the psoas and transversus abdominis muscles. They contain and suspend the ovaries, oviducts and uterine horns together with the associated blood vessels and nerves. The sections of the broad ligaments that attach to the female reproductive tract are the **mesovarium** (ovary), the

mesosalpinx (uterine tube, Fallopian tube, oviduct), the **mesometrium** (uterus) and the **mesovagina** (vagina).

2) **Round ligament of the uterus:** This is a thickened cord of a separate fold of the broad ligament. It is the female homologue of part of the **gubernaculum** (see Section 16.9). In the bitch the round ligament passes through the inguinal canal to insert near the vulva, thereby providing the potential for inguinal hernia.

3) **Proper ligament of the ovary:** The rest of the gubernaculum, extending from the ovary to the paramesonephric duct, becomes the proper ligament of the ovary. The ovaries are secured by proper and suspensory ligaments. The proper ligament attaches the ovary to the cranial extremity of the corresponding uterine horn.

4) The **suspensory ligament** attaches the ovary to the medial surface of the last rib.

### 3.4.4    Pelvic ligaments – male

In the male the gubernaculum extends from the caudal pole of the testis, through the inguinal canal, to the distal scrotum. The proper ligament of the testis attaches the testis to the parietal layer of the peritoneum via the tail of the epididymis (Figure 16.4). See Sections 16.8 and 16.9 for details of the function of the gubernaculum in the descent of the testes.

The gubernacula are paired embryonic ligaments derived from mesenchyme and also called the caudal genital ligaments. They are present in both the male and the female but have more functional significance in the male. In the female they become the ovarian and the round ligaments.

In the immature male the paired gubernacula extend through the inguinal canals to attach to the testes. The proper ligament of the testis attaches the testis to the parietal layer of the peritoneum via the tail of the epididymis (Figure 16.4). The function of the gubernaculum in the descent of the testis is discussed in Section 16.9.

# 4

# The Stomach (Figures 4.1–4.4)

## 4.1   Overview of the Mammalian Stomach

The mammalian stomach is divided into regions that are partly determined by the characteristics of its mucous membrane. The proximal end of the stomach is lined by a region of stratified squamous epithelium similar to that which lines the oesophagus (Figure 4.1); originally termed the oesophageal region but now accepted as truly part of the stomach. The second region, the **cardia**, present only in mammals, is lined by a transitional region of stratified and glandular epithelium. The third compartment is the **fundic** region and is characterised by a lining of simple columnar epithelium containing numerous tubular glands responsible for the production of pepsin (chief cells) and hydrochloric acid (parietal cells).The fourth compartment is the **pyloric** region (some-times referred to as the pyloric antrum) containing branched tubular glands producing a mucoid fluid that has little digestive activity and G cells that produce gastrin, a hor-mone that stimulates secretion by the chief cells and parietal cells. In some species distinct compartments are clearly recognisable in the gross specimen. This is particularly so in the domestic ruminants (see Section 4.2.2), where the region between the oesoph-agus and cardia consists of three compartments, the **rumen, reticulum and omasum**, all lined by stratified squamous epithelium. The **abomasum**, comprising the fundic and pyloric regions, is the equivalent of the glandular stomach of other species. This kind of stomach is known as a **compound stomach**; the stomachs of those species that lack gross compartments are called **simple stomachs**.

## 4.2   Species Variations

### 4.2.1   Horse (Figure 4.1)

The horse's stomach is relatively small, with a capacity of only 5–20 litres depending on the body-size of the horse or pony. It is situated dorsally at the cranial end of the abdom-inal cavity and never extends to the ventral abdominal wall even when full. Its parietal surface faces cranially, dorsally and laterally to the left and is in contact with the left lobe of the liver and diaphragm. The visceral surface is related to the left lobe of the pan-creas, the diaphragmatic flexure and jejunoileum. The small size of the stomach limits

*King's Applied Anatomy of the Abdomen and Pelvis of Domestic Mammals*, First Edition. Geoff Skerritt.
© 2022 John Wiley & Sons Ltd. Published 2022 by John Wiley & Sons Ltd.
Companion website: www.wiley.com/go/skerritt/abdomen

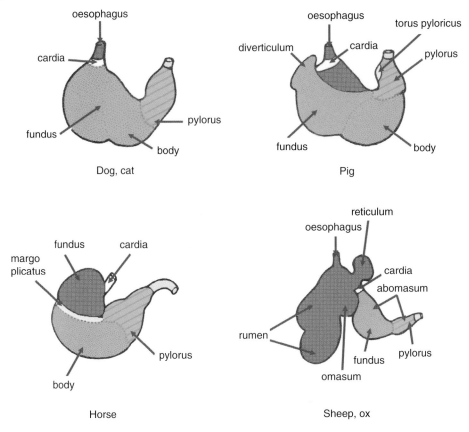

Figure 4.1 The stomachs of the domestic animals. The areas in blue are those parts of the stomach that are lined by a non-glandular, stratified squamous epithelium. The cardiac areas are where the oesophagus enters the stomach in the dog, horse and pig (not shown). In ruminants the cardiac areas are located in the reticulum. In the pig there is a prominent diverticulum of the fundus. In the horse the cardiac zone is very muscular, apparently preventing vomiting. The pyloric zone contains a glandular epithelium (coloured green) and is part of the abomasum in ruminants. The margo plicatus is a distinct ridge separating the glandular (body) and non-glandular areas of the stomach of the horse.

the amount of contents and thereby the quantity of food that can be ingested at any one time. The regions of the stomach are commonly termed as non-glandular (cardia) and glandular (fundic and pyloric). A narrow ridge separating the non-glandular and glandular regions is known as the **margo plicatus**, and the blind-ending part of the fundic region is termed the **saccus caecus**.

The relatively short time that ingesta are in the stomach before being passed through the pyloric sphincter leaves little time (20 minutes) for enzymatic activity, resulting in most digestion occurring in the intestines. No absorption of nutrients occurs in the stomach.

Horses are unable to vomit due to several anatomic differences from most other mammals. The sphincter muscle at the oesophageal entry to the stomach is much better developed than in other animals, and their vomiting reflex is virtually non-existent.

## 4.2.2 Ox (Figures 4.1–4.4)

The stomach of the ox comprises four compartments, three of which are lined by stratified squamous epithelium and termed the rumen, the reticulum and the omasum. The fourth compartment, the abomasum, is lined by a glandular epithelium. The rumen occupies most of the left half of the abdominal cavity. It also extends ventrally and caudally onto the right side. Its long axis extends from the level of the ventral part of the seventh intercostal space to the pelvic inlet. Its relations to the omasum and abomasum are shown in Figures 4.2 and 4.5.

Ruminants (cattle, sheep, goats, camelids, deer, giraffes) are unable to produce enzymes to digest cellulose. However, the ruminoreticulum does contain microbes that promote a microfermentation that breaks down the cellulose. This allows access by the enzymes and hydrochloric acid produced by the glandular epithelium of the abomasum to the nutrients locked within the cellulose barrier. The breakdown of cellulose is further aided by rumination. This is the process of sending the contents of the ruminoreticulum for a second mechanical grinding by the teeth. Known as chewing the **cud**, this practice can occupy the ruminant for up to 8 hours of the day. The omasum is the smallest compartment of the ruminant stomach and is mainly concerned with absorption of water greatly facilitated by the large surface area of the many folds of its inner lining.

The ruminant stomach of the newborn calf is not able to digest the herbivore diet of the adult. In order to digest an early diet of milk, a groove conducts the ingested milk from the cardia directly to the abomasum, bypassing the ruminoreticulum and omasum.

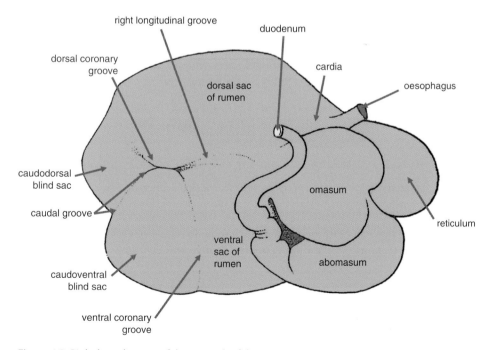

**Figure 4.2** Right lateral aspect of the stomach of the ox.

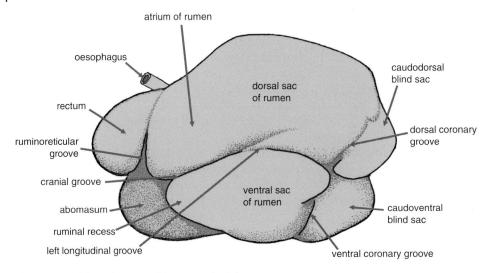

Figure 4.3 Left lateral aspect of the stomach of the ox.

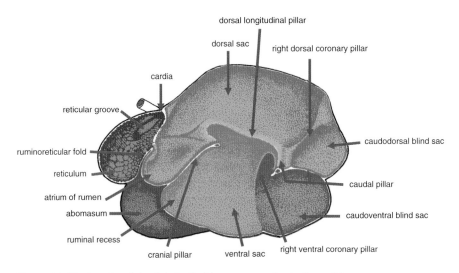

Figure 4.4 The interior of the right half of the rumen and reticulum of the ox.

Muscle fibres in the wall of the groove enable it to close over reflexly and avoid leakage. This important channel is called the **reticular groove** and is often wrongly called the oesophageal groove.

### 4.2.3 Sheep (Figure 4.1)

The stomach of the sheep is similar to that of the ox, although the abomasum is relatively larger. The pylorus is adjacent to the ventral 11th or 12th rib on the right.

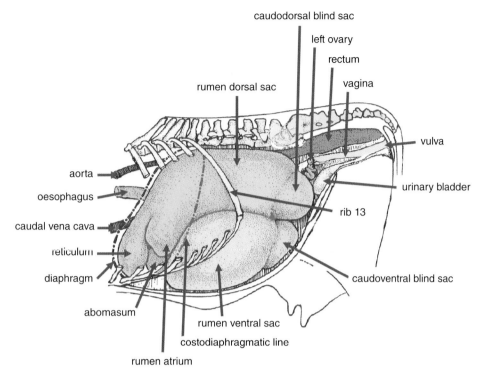

caudodorsal blind sac

left ovary

rectum

rumen dorsal sac

vagina

vulva

aorta

oesophagus

urinary bladder

caudal vena cava

rib 13

reticulum

diaphragm

caudoventral blind sac

abomasum

rumen ventral sac

costodiaphragmatic line

rumen atrium

Figure 4.5 Left lateral aspect of the gastrointestinal tract of the ox, in situ. The rumen, as shown, is not completely full and consequently has not extended into the pelvic inlet. The uterine cornu and left ovary are therefore visible.

### 4.2.4 Pig (Figure 4.1)

The stomach of the pig is relatively large compared with that of the horse. When moderately full it lies entirely within the thoracic cage (Figure 5.4), mainly on the left side. The parietal surface is in contact with the liver and dorsal region of the diaphragm. The visceral surface is related to the spleen on the left and to the coils of the ascending colon (Figure 6.3). When fully distended the stomach makes extensive contact with the abdominal wall, not only ventrally and on the left but on the right side also. Unlike the simple stomachs of the other species, the pig possesses a **diverticulum** of the fundus that is directed caudally and ventrally. The diverticulum is lined by a glandular mucosa, although its developmental origin is the same as part of the rumen.

### 4.2.5 Dog

The empty stomach lies entirely within the caudal part of the thoracic cage, in contact with the left region of the visceral (caudal) surface of the liver. It is fixed in position at the cardia by the diaphragm and at the lesser curvature by the lesser omentum. The full stomach extends caudally well beyond the thoracic cage and makes extensive contact with the ventral body wall. In doing so it tends to displace the intestinal mass and the spleen caudodorsally. The stomach is particularly distensible in puppies.

The stomach of the dog is frequently examined by endoscopy for the investigation of vomiting and the presence of foreign bodies. In this procedure the location of the **angular incisura** in the lesser curvature of the stomach (Figure 4.1) of the dog is an important landmark for endoscopy.

## 4.3   Clinical Conditions

### 4.3.1   Horse

**Gastric ulceration:** Erosion and even perforation of the gastric mucosa is of high incidence. The factors involved are multifactorial with stress, exercise and diet all of proven involvement. Production of the hydrochloric acid secreted by parietal cells is stimulated by gastrin, histamine and acetylcholine.

   **Gastric impaction:** This is not a common condition and tends to occur alongside a recurrence of colic (see Section 6.3). The retention of gastric contents occurs when the feed swells or when there are dental problems affecting the ability to chew the food adequately.

   Gastric dilatation and rupture can be a sequel to impaction or to small or large intestinal obstruction. Rupture usually occurs along the greater curvature of the stomach.

### 4.3.2   Ox

**Vagus indigestion (see Section 11.5):** This is a chronic syndrome of indigestion in ruminants but mainly cattle. Various causes have been suggested, but the condition seems most likely to be due to damage to branches of the vagus nerves as a consequence of traumatic reticuloperitonitis. Loss of appetite, reduced milk yield, weight and condition loss and abdominal distention are clinical signs. The prognosis is poor.

   **Displaced abomasum:** The abomasum is fairly mobile, being only loosely anchored by the greater omentum (see Section 3.2 and 3.3). During pregnancy the position of the abomasum becomes altered by the presence of the pregnant uterus. Displacement can be either to the left or right although more commonly to the left, where it becomes trapped ventral to the rumen. Accumulation of gas and obstruction to movement of ingesta occur with a left displacement. The situation is more serious with a right displacement since haemostasis and damage to the vagal nerves are likely to result from torsion of the abomasum. Loss of appetite and condition in a recently calved cow are usual indicators of displaced abomasum, and diagnosis is confirmed by auscultation with a stethoscope when a characteristic sound is heard.

   **Bloat:** This condition can occur as a result of engorgement of lush pasture. Accumulation of fermentation gas leads to distention of the rumen with resulting pressure on the heart and lungs. Death can result without emergency attention usually involving the insertion of a trocar and cannula into the rumen in the left dorsal flank.

### 4.3.3   Sheep

**Bloat:** Although not as common as in cattle, the sheep's stomach is susceptible to bloat. Internal parasites in the gastrointestinal tract can be responsible for loss of condition.

### 4.3.4  Pig

**Gastric ulceration:** Growing pigs are the most susceptible to ulceration of the stomach. Erosion and ulceration of the mucosa in the oesophageal of the stomach can occur for a variety of reasons, e.g. too small particle size of the diet.

**Gastric torsion:** Overfeeding and large amounts of wet feed can be causative factors of gastric torsion. Swollen abdomen and sudden death (2–3 hours) are presenting signs. The torsion is often not restricted to the stomach but can involve the intestines as well. Dilatation of the stomach and congestion of blood vessels are usual findings at post-mortem.

### 4.3.5  Dog

**Gastritis:** Inflammatory conditions of the stomach are common in the dog. The causes are many including contaminated food, ingested irritants and toxic plants. The pathogenesis involves damage to the mucosa and an inflammatory response. The clinical signs are vomiting, anorexia and depression.

**Gastric dilatation and volvulus (GDV):** This condition is of frequent occurrence in large breed dogs, e.g. Great Dane, Irish Setter, Gordon Setter, Weimaraner and St. Bernard. The mortality rate is high (33.3% in one study). The cause is not clear but there does seem to be a predilection in barrel-chested individuals of the breeds above and other large breeds. Stress and overeating have been identified as possible causes but not proven. The pathogenesis of GDV involves gastric dilatation followed by gastric rotation leading to ischaemia and necrosis of the mucosal and smooth muscle layers of the stomach wall. Prompt shock therapy and surgical correction of the rotation are the necessary procedures.

**Foreign bodies:** The ingestion of foreign bodies is frequent in dogs and involves a variety of objects. The author once removed nine golf balls from the stomach of a German Shepherd! Vomiting is the most likely clinical sign of a gastric foreign body. Palpation rarely detects an object in the stomach, and radiography depends on the nature of the foreign body. Longhaired cats often ingest hair that may accumulate as a hairball in the stomach. Surgical removal of the foreign body is usually indicated.

# 5

# The Small Intestines

## 5.1 Duodenum, Jejunum and Ileum

The duodenum is the first section of the small intestine. It is located dorsally and begins on the right side at the pylorus, the exit sphincter of the stomach. The duodenum receives **chyme**, a mixture of partially digested stomach contents and gastric acid. Ascending and descending limbs of the duodenum are recognised, but the division into the three sections of the small intestine are difficult to determine.

The small intestine is the principal site for chemical digestion of nutrients. Although most of digestive function is provided by the enzymes produced and secreted by the pancreas, the mucosal cells of the small intestine also make a contribution. Brunner's glands are present in man within the duodenal mucosa but not in the domestic mammals. They produce bicarbonate, which neutralises the gastric acid that has passed through the pylorus.

Histologically the small intestine comprises an outer serosa (visceral peritoneum), two layers of smooth muscle (inner circular and outer longitudinal), a submucosa and a mucosa. The internal surface area of the mucosa is increased by the presence of finger-like projections called villi and further minute projections called microvilli. This arrangement effectively increases the area for absorption of the products of digestion. In the sub-mucosal areas of the small intestine are located the intestinal crypts (**crypts of Lieberkuhn**) containing a variety of cells with different functions. These cells include the **Paneth cells**, whose function seems to be the protection of stem cells against bacterial invasion. The stem cells are capable of self-renewal of the intestinal crypt cells.

The myenteric plexus (**Auerbach's plexus**) (see Section 11.4.5) lies between the muscle layers and comprises both sympathetic and parasympathetic unmyelinated fibres and cell bodies; it innervates the muscle of the intestine.

All species possess small aggregations of lymphoid tissue mainly in the distal section of the ileum but sometimes located in the distal jejunum. These are the **Peyer's patches** and consist of B lymphocyte follicles, enterocytes and M cells; they function as primary lymphoid tissue entrapping foreign particles and destroying potentially pathogenic microorganisms. M cells transport antigens from the lumen of the intestine to the lymphoid tissue. Enterocytes are columnar epithelial cells that absorb nutrients, electrolytes and water.

*King's Applied Anatomy of the Abdomen and Pelvis of Domestic Mammals*, First Edition. Geoff Skerritt.
© 2022 John Wiley & Sons Ltd. Published 2022 by John Wiley & Sons Ltd.
Companion website: www.wiley.com/go/skerritt/abdomen

Most of the enzymes that digest nutrients in the small intestine are secreted by the pancreas and enter the duodenum via the pancreatic ducts. These are variable (see Section 7.6), but the main duct is more constant and opens into the cranial duodenum with the common bile duct. When present the accessory pancreatic duct opens into the descending duodenum.

## 5.2 Species Variations

### 5.2.1 Horse (Figure 5.1 and 5.2)

The duodenum is fairly firmly fixed by the mesoduodenum to the liver and the right dorsal colon. Immediately after the pylorus it turns sharply cranially through the sigmoid flexure and then caudally at the caudal flexure. The remainder of the small intestine is very variable in position, lying in numerous coils with the small (descending) colon, chiefly in the left dorsal part of the abdomen from the stomach to the pelvic inlet.

Initially the descending duodenum is related to the right kidney and the base of the caecum. It passes laterally and caudally around the base of the caecum and then crosses the midline. The ascending duodenum passes cranially on the left side, reaching the left kidney; there it continues into the jejunum. The small intestine of the horse is about 20 metres long.

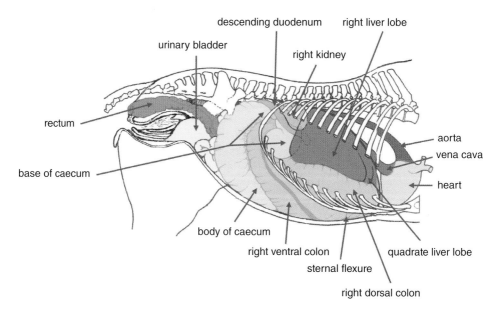

Figure 5.1 Right aspect of the gastrointestinal tract of a mare in situ.

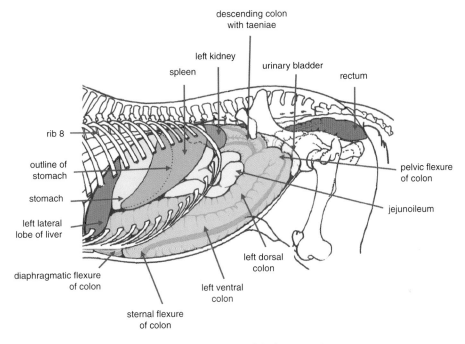

Figure 5.2 Left aspect of the gastrointestinal tract of the horse, in situ.

### 5.2.2 Ox (Figure 5.3)

The small intestine is up to 40 metres in length and 5–6 cm in diameter depending on the size of the animal. The duodenum is about 1 metre long and begins at the pylorus adjacent to the ventral end of the 10th rib on the right side. The diameter of the small intestine is 5–6 cm. The coils of the small intestine mostly occupy the ventral part of the right flank.

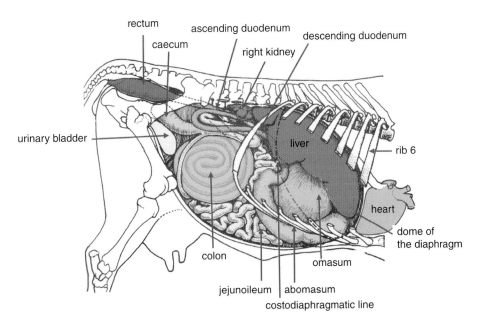

Figure 5.3 Right lateral aspect of the gastrointestinal tract of the ox, in situ

### 5.2.3 Sheep

The pylorus is located on the right side opposite the ventral end of the ninth rib. After passing dorsally and cranially to the visceral surface of the liver, the duodenum makes an S-shaped curve to reach the cranial pole of the right kidney. The duodenum then passes caudally to the level of the tuber coxae, where it turns cranially at the iliac flexure and, at the level of the right kidney, becomes the jejunum. The coils of he jejunoileum reach the caecocolic junction on the medial side at the level of the last rib.

### 5.2.4 Pig (Figure 5.4)

The stomach is fairly distended and contacts the body wall.

The duodenum is related to the liver and kidneys as in the dog. The jejunum lies mainly in the right caudal quadrant of the abdominal cavity but extends into the caudoventral region on the left.

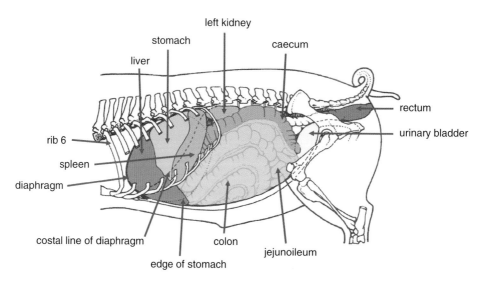

Figure 5.4 Left lateral aspect of the gastrointestinal tract of the pig, in situ.

### 5.2.5 Dog (Figure 5.5 and 5.6)

The small intestine of the dog is a narrow tube about two and a half times the length of the dog. The duodenum is relatively fixed in position by the short mesoduodenum. The cranial part of the duodenum is short and leaves the pylorus to lie across the liver from left to right; it is related to ribs 9 and 10 and lies in contact with the upper right flank. The descending duodenum passes caudally from the liver and on the ventral surface of the right kidney almost to the pelvic inlet. The ascending duodenum starts just cranial to the pelvic inlet and runs cranially on the left side of the abdomen, ventral to the descending colon and left kidney. The descending and ascending parts are in a V shape (Figure 2.1).

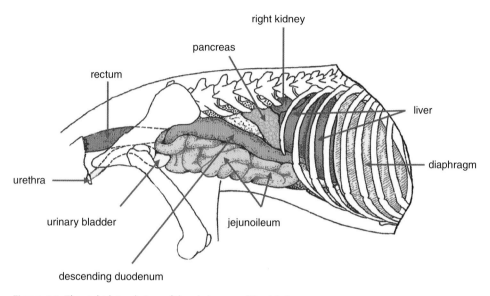

Figure 5.5 The right lateral view of the abdomen of the bitch.

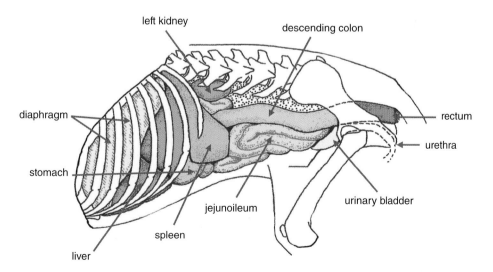

Figure 5.6 The left lateral view of the abdomen of the dog.

The jejunoileum is long and very mobile, in contrast to the duodenum and colon, which are short and relatively fixed in position. The jejunoileum is separated from the ventral and lateral body walls by the greater omentum (see Section 3.2).

## 5.3 Clinical Conditions

### 5.3.1 Horse (Figure 5.2)

The small intestine of the horse is susceptible to a variety of inflammatory causes. Bacterial and parasitic infections can be responsible for a serious onset of enteritis. The resulting abdominal pain can be due to torsion of the intestine, and death can result if urgent treatment is delayed. This condition is referred to as colic (see Section 6.3).

### 5.3.2 Ox

**Johne's disease:** This is the name given to a disease of the small intestine of ruminants. It is caused by the bacterium *Mycobacterium paratuberculosis* and is seen most frequently in cattle but can affect non-ruminant species. The bacterium invades the small intestine and is transported by the M cells to the Peyer's patches of the ileum (see Section 5.1). Here it is captured by macrophages, but rather than being rendered harmless, the usual function of the macrophages, the bacteria promote an overgrowth of lymphocytes. As a result, there is thickening of the intestine wall with a serious obstruction to absorption of nutrients. Affected animals lose weight, suffer diarrhoea and die.

### 5.3.3 Sheep

**Johne's disease:** This disease is less common in sheep than in cattle. The pathogen is again *Mycobacterium paratuberculosis* (*M. johnei*). In sheep, unlike in cattle, diarrhoea is not usually a feature. The presenting signs are weight loss and loss of condition. The pathogenesis is the same as in cattle, i.e. thickening of the small intestine wall with resulting malabsorption.

### 5.3.4 Pig

**Transmissible gastroenteritis:** This is a coronavirus infection causing vomiting and diarrhoea in pigs of any age. The virus destroys epithelial villi in the jejunoileum, resulting in malabsorption and dehydration.

### 5.3.5 Dog

**Canine parvovirus:** Canine parvovirus infection is a highly contagious and virulent infection of dogs and some non-domestic mammals. Two forms of the disease are recognised – intestinal and cardiac. Puppies of certain breeds (e.g. Dobermanns and Rottweilers) are particularly susceptible, and death can occur within 48 hours without treatment. The clinical signs are usually sudden onset of vomiting and diarrhoea accompanied by leucopenia and dehydration. In the cardiac form myocarditis develops and can be followed by sudden death. In the intestinal form the virus has a particular affinity for actively dividing cells, e.g. lymphoid tissue, bone marrow and the cells of the intestinal crypts.

**Haemorrhagic gastroenteritis:** This condition is characterised by an acute onset of haemorrhagic diarrhoea and vomiting. Small and toy breed dogs under 5 years of age seem especially susceptible. The cause is unknown, but a Clostridial infection has been suspected. The principal lesion is a haemorrhagic inflammation and necrosis of the intestines. Involvement of the stomach is minimal, and the lesion affects the large intestine more than the small one.

**Foreign body:** A variety of foreign bodies may be swallowed by dogs and cats. Common items are toys, bones, socks and fishhooks. The clinical signs relate to intestinal obstruction, i.e. abdominal discomfort, vomiting, loss of appetite. Palpation and radiography may lead to a prompt diagnosis.

**Malabsorption:** The pancreatic enzymes convert many of the nutrients presented at the intestinal mucosa into simpler compounds that are able to cross the enterocyte barrier and enter the bloodstream on their way to the liver. However, if the pancreatic enzymes are deficient, this process of aided absorption is severely retarded. This situation is labelled exocrine pancreatic insufficiency (EPI) and occurs in dogs. Malabsorption can also be a result of small intestinal bacterial overgrowth (SIBO). German Shepherd Dogs are the breed most commonly affected by these conditions, which may occur singly or together.

**Intussception:** A variety of causes can be responsible for a telescoping of the intestine, e.g. intestinal parasites, bacterial or viral infections, foreign bodies, intestinal tumours and dietary changes. Usually, the intussception involves peristaltic entry of a proximal segment into a static distal segment. Intussceptions occur most commonly in the jejunum and in puppies. Diagnosis is by palpation or radiography in a dog or cat with sudden onset of vomiting, diarrhoea, abdominal pain and straining to defaecate. Any delay in treatment rapidly results in haemostasis and tissue necrosis. Early surgical manipulation may be successful, but resection and anastomosis may be necessary.

# 6

# The Large Intestine

## 6.1 Overview

The large intestine comprises the **colon, caecum, rectum** and **anal canal**. Its primary functions are the absorption of water from its contents and the voiding of waste matter via the anus. However, there is considerable variation amongst mammals in the anatomy of the large intestine in relation to the diet. Ruminants digest a herbivorous diet primarily in the stomach, whereas the horse digests its herbivorous diet in the large intestine. The dog and cat are carnivores and digest their food in the stomach and small intestine. The pig is omnivorous, and its digestive tract anatomy and function are similar to that of the dog.

The caecum is a diverticulum of the proximal colon. There is great variation in the anatomy of the caecum of the domestic mammals. As a rule, the caecum of herbivores is large and that of carnivores is small. This difference is related to the storage and breakdown of cellulose by bacteria that occurs in the caecum of herbivores. The appendix is an appendage to the caecum in humans but absent in the domestic animals; it is usually 6–9 cm in length and contains lymphoid tissue.

The colon is divided into ascending, transverse and descending sections in all the domestic mammals. The descending colon is narrower than the other parts and is continuous with the rectum. All carnivores possess two **perianal sacs** located one either side between the internal and external anal sphincters (see Figure 18.6). The sacs are oval-shaped and 0.5–1.0 cm in diameter and store the sebaceous secretion of glands in the lining of the sacs. The glands are coiled, tubular and apocrine. The secretion is a strong-smelling territory marker and commonly becomes impacted in dogs when it requires manual expression.

## 6.2 Species Variations

### 6.2.1 Horse (Figures 5.1, 5.2 and 6.1)

The **caecum** resembles a gigantic comma, with the base dorsal in position and the body and the apex curving ventrally and cranially to reach the sternum. Except for the apex, it lies to the right of the midline. The base is firmly attached to the right sublumbar

*King's Applied Anatomy of the Abdomen and Pelvis of Domestic Mammals*, First Edition. Geoff Skerritt.
© 2022 John Wiley & Sons Ltd. Published 2022 by John Wiley & Sons Ltd.
Companion website: www.wiley.com/go/skerritt/abdomen

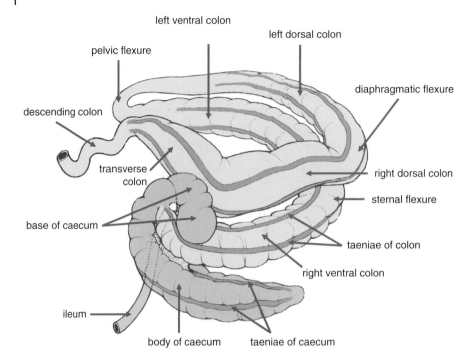

Figure 6.1 Caecum and ascending colon of the horse. The organs are viewed from the right side and from a slightly dorsal position. The body and apex of the caecum have been pulled ventrally and somewhat to the right.

region and to the right kidney. The descending duodenum passes around the base. The apex and much of the body lie on the abdominal floor, between the right ventral and left ventral colons. The caecum has four longitudinal muscle bands.

The **large (ascending) colon** has four divisions:

1) **Right ventral colon:** extends from the base of the caecum at about the ventral part of the last rib, along the costal arch and abdominal floor to the **xiphoid cartilage**. There it turns sharply as the sternal flexure. Four longitudinal muscle bands (**taeniae coli**) continue those of the caecum.

2) **Left ventral colon:** passes back along the abdominal floor, on the left of the caecum, to the general vicinity of the pelvic inlet. Here it bends sharply dorsally and cranially as the pelvic flexure. The pelvic flexure is very variable in its position and can cross to the right flank. There are again four longitudinal muscle bands. Beyond the pelvic flexure, the calibre of the colon is much reduced.

3) **Left dorsal colon:** much reduced in calibre, this runs cranially, lying dorsal or lateral to the left ventral colon, to reach the diaphragm and left lobe of the liver, and there turns back and to the right as the diaphragmatic flexure. Starting at the pelvic flexure, one longitudinal band is present, and this can be palpated per rectum.

4) **Right dorsal colon:** lies entirely within the thoracic cage. It passes caudally, dorsal to the right ventral colon. At the base of the caecum it turns medially, very close to

the stomach and liver, and continues as the transverse colon. Three longitudinal muscle bands are present.

**The transverse colon** crosses from the right to the left side, cranial to the root of the mesentery. Its calibre is constricted, compared with the right dorsal colon.

**The small colon** (descending colon) begins at the end of the transverse colon, ventral to the left kidney and immediately caudal to the **saccus caecus** of the stomach. It mingles with the small intestine, occupying a similar position, i.e. mainly in the left dorsal part of the abdominal cavity. Its calibre is considerably less than that of the ascending colon. It has two longitudinal muscle bands and two rows of sacculations, and these features distinguish it from the small intestine.

### 6.2.2   Ox (Figures 4.5, 5.3 and 6.2)

The **caecum** extends caudodorsally in the upper part of the right flank. Its blind extremity terminates at the right side of the pelvic inlet, where it is related to the rectum dorsally and the urinary bladder ventrally. The coils of the **colon** lie in the right caudal quadrant of the abdominal cavity. The general relations of the proximal loop, spiral loop and distal loop are shown in Figure 6.2.

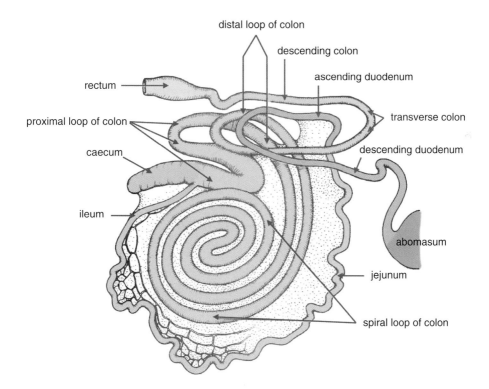

**Figure 6.2** Semi-diagrammatic right lateral view of the intestines of the ox to show the proximal loop, the spiral loop and the distal loop of the ascending colon.

### 6.2.3 Sheep

The large intestine of the sheep is very similar to that of the ox. The **caecum** is about 10 inches long and 2 inches wide. The **colon** is about 15 feet long, and its diameter narrows distally.

### 6.2.4 Pig (Figures 5.4 and 6.3)

The caecocolic junction is dorsal and, on the left, related to the caudal pole of the left kidney. The **caecum** is directed ventrally and caudally, covering the caudal aspect of the coils of the ascending colon. It lies in contact with the left abdominal wall. The apex often lies on the ventral body wall, more or less in the midline.

The **ascending colon** forms a conical spiral. The direction taken by the axis of the spiral varies with the fullness of the stomach, but essentially it points ventrally and slightly to the left. The effect of this is to bring the spiral colon into extensive contact with the left abdominal wall as in Figure 6.3 The transverse colon lies in the usual position. The descending colon passes straight to the pelvic inlet close to the dorsal midline.

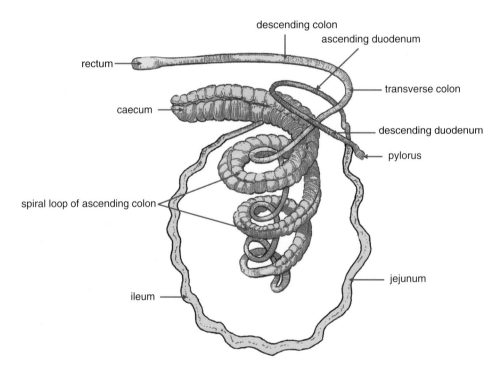

Figure 6.3 Diagram of the intestines of the pig as viewed from the right side.

### 6.2.5  Dog (Figures 5.5 and 5.6)

The **caecum** lies within the V of the duodenal loop, ventral to the right transverse processes of lumbar vertebrae two to four. It is related to the descending duodenum and the right kidney.

The **ascending colon** extends cranially on the right side of the abdominal roof, between the descending duodenum on its right and the small intestinal mass ventrally on its left. The **transverse colon** runs from right to left, cranial to the cranial mesenteric artery passing caudodorsally to the stomach. The **descending colon** lies against the upper part of the left flank covered by the greater omentum. It is related to the left kidney and the ascending duodenum.

## 6.3  Clinical Conditions

**Colic** is a serious and potentially fatal clinical condition of horses. It is characterised by evidence of anxiety and abdominal pain. There are several types of colic ranging from excessive gas accumulation in the gastrointestinal tract to obstruction or strangulation. The cause of colic may be inflammation of the gastrointestinal tract or ulceration of the gut mucosa. Although the name suggests that this is a condition of the colon, colic can involve any part of the gastrointestinal tract. Severe cases may require urgent surgical intervention to correct the cause, e.g. strangulation, whereas less severe cases may be managed conservatively with spasmolytic agents and anti-inflammatory drugs.

Both acute and chronic **colitis** occur commonly in the dog. Acute colitis is usually due to the ingestion of some infectious or contaminated material. Bacterial or parasitic causes may be detected and are responsible for profuse and watery diarrhoea, often including mucus and blood. Chronic colitis presents as a persistent or recurrent diarrhoea that is difficult to define. Due to the important function of the colon in promoting resorption of water, dehydration is often a significant feature of colitis and necessitates fluid replacement.

Tumours of the colon occur but are not common in dogs and are usually benign polyps.

# 7

# The Liver and Pancreas

## 7.1 The Liver (Figure 7.1)

The liver is an accessory digestive organ found only in vertebrates. It has many functions (Zakim and Boyer suggest as many as 500 in *Hepatology: A Textbook of Liver Disease*); herewith the more important ones:

1) Production of bile, an alkaline fluid that is involved in the breakdown of ingested fat; it contains cholesterol and bile acids
2) Protein synthesis, e.g. hormones and enzymes
3) Regulation of glycogen storage
4) Decomposition of red blood cells.

## 7.2 Anatomy of the Liver

The liver comprises four lobes; left, right, caudate and quadrate as listed in the *Nomina Anatomica Veterinaria* (*NAV*), although Sisson and Grossman also identify a 'middle' lobe that includes the quadrate lobe in the horse. The **left** and **right lobes** are subdivided into medial and lateral divisions. The **quadrate lobe** lies in the medial plane between the right medial and the left medial/lateral lobes. The gall bladder is located between the quadrate lobe medially and the right medial lobe laterally. The **caudate lobe** comprises the **papillary process** and the **caudate process**. The papillary process is covered by the lesser omentum and the caudate process is in close proximity to the cranial pole of the right kidney.

Between the right and left lobes is the **hilus** of the liver; it is the location of the bile duct, blood vessels and nerves entering and leaving the liver, and it is also termed the porta of the liver. The nerves and arteries enter the porta dorsally, the bile duct exits ventrally and the hepatic portal vein enters the porta centrally.

The falciform ligament (see Section 3.4.1) separates the left and right lobes. It is a remnant of the ventral mesentery, which extended to the umbilicus from the liver and diaphragm. The parietal surface of the liver is in contact with the diaphragm, and the visceral surface contacts the cranial abdominal viscera. The liver lies almost entirely within the costal arch and is not normally palpable. The visceral surface bears impressions of the adjacent abdominal viscera.

*King's Applied Anatomy of the Abdomen and Pelvis of Domestic Mammals*, First Edition. Geoff Skerritt.
© 2022 John Wiley & Sons Ltd. Published 2022 by John Wiley & Sons Ltd.
Companion website: www.wiley.com/go/skerritt/abdomen

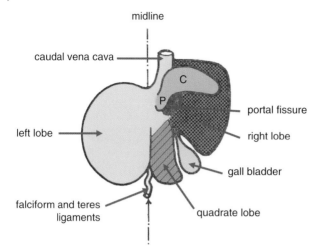

Figure 7.1 Diagram of the caudal view showing the visceral surfaces of a typical mammalian liver. Figures 7.2–7.4 illustrate the species variations. There are four main lobes; the left and right hepatic lobes are subdivided into medial and lateral lobes. The caudate lobe (C) comprises the caudal and papillary processes (P). The quadrate lobe lies adjacent to the gall bladder.

## 7.3   Histology of the Liver

The liver lobes consist of hexagonal-shaped **hepatic lobules**, each radiating from a central vein. The basic cells are the hepatocytes, which surround sinusoids. Blood enters the sinusoids from both portal venules (about 75%) and hepatic arterioles. Following complex chemical exchanges, the blood leaves the sinusoids to enter the central veins, which drain via hepatic veins to the caudal vena cava.

The hepatic lobules also contain **bile canaliculi** that receive bile secreted by the hepatocytes. The bile drains to the common bile duct via progressively larger bile ducts.

## 7.4   The Gall Bladder

The **cystic duct** drains bile from the gall bladder and is joined by the hepatic ducts to form the **common bile duct**, the passage to the duodenum. There are no valves in the bile ducts so that bile may flow in either direction. Bile can flow via the cystic duct to be concentrated and stored in the gall bladder. The common bile duct empties into the duodenum at the major duodenal papilla, a short distance from the pylorus.

The presence of food containing fat within the gastrointestinal tract stimulates the secretion of the hormone **cholecystokinin** (pancreozymin) by inclusion cells (specialised fibroblasts). This hormone causes contraction of the gall bladder wall and release of bile into the duodenum. The bile emulsifies fats in the ingesta, thereby facilitating absorption.

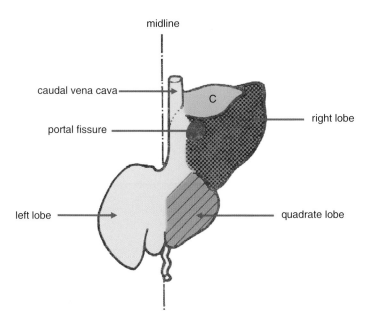

Figure 7.2  The liver of the horse. The left lobe is subdivided and the papillary lobe is absent. There is no gall bladder.

## 7.5  Species Variations

### 7.5.1  Horse (Figure 7.2)

The cranial surface of the liver is closely applied to the diaphragm, mostly to the right of the midline. Its most dorsal part is at the level of the right kidney, and its most ventral part is 7–10 cm from the abdominal floor opposite the seventh or eighth rib. Its most cranial part is at the level of the ventral third of the sixth or seventh rib. The horse does **not** have a gall bladder.

### 7.5.2  Ruminants (Figure 7.3)

The liver of the domestic ruminants lies to the right of the midline, except a small part of which lies ventral to the oesophageal notch. The diaphragmatic surface is in extensive contact with the diaphragm. The visceral surface is related to the atrium of the rumen and to the reticulum, omasum and the cranial part of the duodenum. Dorsally the liver is embedded against the right kidney.

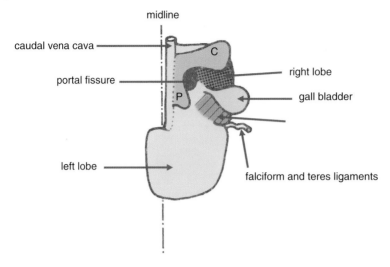

**Figure 7.3** The liver of ruminants. The liver is almost entirely displaced to the right. The umbilical fissure is deeper in the sheep than the ox and the gall bladder does not project so far. The caudate lobe is smaller in the sheep than in the ox.

### 7.5.3 Pig (Figure 7.4)

The parietal surface of the liver fits the dome of the diaphragm. The visceral surface is in contact with the stomach. Unlike all the other domestic mammals there is no contact with the right kidney. There is therefore no renal impression.

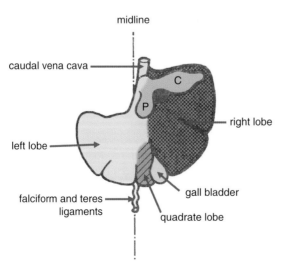

**Figure 7.4** Diagram of the liver of the dog, cat and pig. The right and left lobes are subdivided into medial and lateral lobes.

## 7.5.4 Dog and Cat (Figure 7.4)

The liver lies almost entirely within the thoracic cage. Cranially its parietal surface is in contact with the diaphragm. Caudally its visceral surface is related on the left to the stomach and on the right to the duodenum, right kidney and pancreas.

## 7.6 The Pancreas

The pancreas is a bilobed, lobulated, elongated gland located in the right, dorsal abdomen. The right lobe lies in contact with the descending duodenum and the left lobe lies in the dorsal leaf of the greater omentum (see Section 3.2).

The pancreas has both an endocrine and an exocrine function. The **pancreatic islets** (islets of Langerhans) produce the endocrine secretions, insulin (beta cells), glucagon (alpha cells), somatostatin (delta cells) and pancreatic polypeptide (gamma cells), and their function is mainly the regulation of blood sugar levels. The exocrine function is the secretion of pancreatic juice containing digestive enzymes for action on carbohydrates, proteins and fats within the duodenum. The alkalinity of the pancreatic juice is maintained by the production of bicarbonate, which neutralises the acidic gastric juice.

The pancreas has two excretory ducts in the horse and dog. The **pancreatic duct** is the larger in the dog and is located on the ventral side of the duodenum in close association to the opening of the common bile duct. The **accessory pancreatic duct** enters the duodenum on its dorsal side. The ruminants and the pig have only one pancreatic duct (it is the accessory duct that is present).

## 7.7 Clinical Conditions of the Liver and Pancreas

**Hepatitis** is an inflammatory condition of the liver. In dogs infectious canine hepatitis is caused by Canine mastadenovirus A (formerly called Canine adenovirus 1 [CAV-1]). The clinical signs of pyrexia, jaundice, vomiting and signs of encephalopathy are typical of canine hepatitis and usually resolve after a brief illness. Most dogs receive an effective vaccine. In the large domestic animals, hepatitis is usually due to ingested plant toxins, e.g. ragwort.

**Portosystemic shunts (PSSs)** are of regular occurrence in dogs and cats. A PSS is the presence of vascularity that bypasses the liver, allowing blood from the hepatic portal vein to go directly to the caudal vena cava. This abnormality results in the inability of the liver to deal directly with toxins, proteins, hormones and nutrients absorbed by the intestines. Most PSSs are congenital in origin and result in neurological signs, e.g. seizures, unsteadiness and blindness. Surgical treatment of PSSs usually involves complete or partial occlusion of the abnormal vessel.

Cattle, sheep, deer and horses may be infected with **liver fluke** (*Fasciola hepatica*). This is a parasite with the snail (*Galba truncatula*) as the intermediate host. The domestic animals ingest the larvae when grazing pasture during the autumn. The oval-shaped flukes, up to 3 cm long, penetrate the gut wall and migrate in the bloodstream to the liver. Affected animals lose condition, become anaemic and develop 'bottle jaw' – oedema under the mandible. Treatment usually involves the oral administration of an anthelmintic drug (e.g. triclabendazole).

Inadequate production of insulin by beta cells in the pancreas islets results in inefficient metabolism of sugars, fats and proteins. This condition is called **diabetes mellitus** and occurs in dogs and cats. Overweight individuals and those with inflammation of the pancreas are predisposed to developing diabetes. Long-term therapy with corticosteroid drugs can result in iatrogenic diabetes. Diagnosis of diabetes is made by finding sugar in the urine and an increase in blood sugar. Diabetes is usually treated by the regular (once or twice daily) subcutaneous administration of insulin.

# 8

# Arteries of the Abdomen and Pelvis (Figures 8.1–8.3)

The major arterial supply to the abdomen and pelvis is provided by the dorsal aorta. This arterial trunk leaves the left ventricle of the heart and bends towards the diaphragm. The right subclavian artery and the brachiocephalic trunk branch off the aorta in a cranial direction, and the aorta bends caudally. The brachiocephalic trunk gives rise to the right subclavian artery and the two common carotid arteries. The aorta lies dorsally in the thorax, just ventral to the thoracic vertebrae, and passes caudally to the diaphragm. The aorta perforates the diaphragm at the **aortic hiatus**, a fibrous ring located dorsally immediately ventral to the L3/L4 vertebrae. The aortic hiatus lies between the left and right crura of the diaphragm. The hiatus is further reinforced by the sublumbar muscles (e.g. psoas muscles).

The diaphragm is also perforated by the **oesophageal hiatus** and the **caudal caval foramen**. The former is located between the crura but further away from the tendinous origins and is not supported by the sublumbar muscles. The oesophageal hiatus is reinforced by collagen fibres and must be capable of expansion to allow swallowing; nevertheless, this is a weak point with the risk of herniation. The caudal caval foramen is further ventral, perforating the tendinous centre of the diaphragm.

The abdominal aorta is displaced slightly to the left by the caudal vena cava and lies along the roof of the abdomen in a furrow between the left and right psoas muscles. The abdominal aorta ends caudally at the level of the last lumbar vertebra, where it divides into the pair of **external iliac** arteries.

Between the diaphragm and the caudal bifurcation the abdominal aorta gives origin to a succession of both paired and midline arterial branches.

## 8.1  The Branches of the Abdominal Aorta

The listing and description of the major abdominal arteries given below is for the dog with added notes of important species variations. The coeliac, cranial mesenteric and caudal mesenteric arteries are single; all the other branches of the aorta are paired.

*King's Applied Anatomy of the Abdomen and Pelvis of Domestic Mammals*, First Edition. Geoff Skerritt.
© 2022 John Wiley & Sons Ltd. Published 2022 by John Wiley & Sons Ltd.
Companion website: www.wiley.com/go/skerritt/abdomen

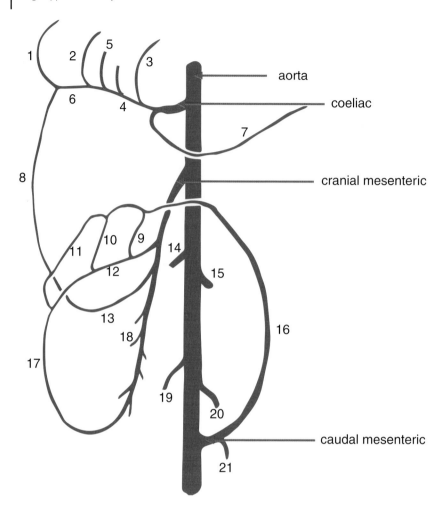

**Figure 8.1** Ventral view diagram of the main arteries of the abdomen of the dog. 1 = right gastroepiploic; 2 = right gastric; 3 = left gastric; 4 = common hepatic; 5 = proper hepatic; 6 = gastroduodenal; 7 = splenic; 8 = cranial pancreaticoduodenal; 9 = middle colic; 10 = right colic; 11 = colic branch; 12 = common colic; 13 = caudal pancreaticoduodenal; 14 = right renal; 15 = left renal; 16 = left colic; 17 = ileocecocolic; 18 = jejunal; 19 = right testicular/ovarian; 20 = left testicular/ovarian; 21 = cranial rectal.

### 8.1.1   Coeliac artery

This is the first visceral branch of the abdominal aorta. It is surrounded by a large plexus of nerves and the two coeliac ganglia (coeliacomesenteric plexus) together with numerous lymphatic vessels. The coeliac artery arises unpaired between the crura of the diaphragm and is only about 2 cm long. Usually it trifurcates into the **common hepatic** artery, **left gastric** artery and **splenic** artery. The common hepatic artery lies in a groove of the pancreas before it splits into several proper hepatic arteries supplying the liver parenchyma. The left of these hepatic arteries supplies the left lateral, left medial and quadrate lobes as well as a **cystic branch** to the gall bladder.

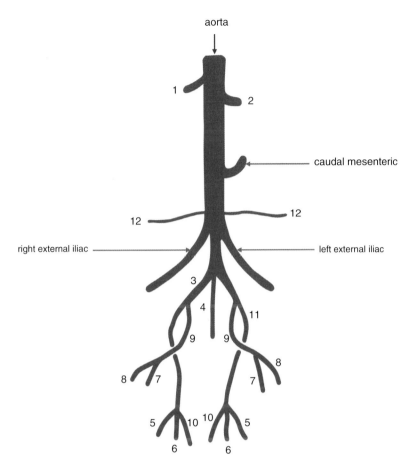

Figure 8.2 Diagram of the arteries of the pelvis of the dog. 1 = right testicular; 2 = left testicular/ovarian; 3 = right internal iliac; 4 = median sacral; 5 = caudal gluteal; 6 = perineal; 7 = internal pududental; 8 = urogenital; 9 = visceral internal iliac; 10 = iliolumbar; 11 = parietal internal iliac; 12 = deep circumflex iliac.

The common hepatic artery becomes the gastroduodenal artery before terminating as the right gastroepiploic and cranial pancreaticoduodenal arteries. Both the numerous gastric and epiploic branches make numerous anastomoses in the stomach wall and the great omentum.

The splenic artery is a vessel of comparatively large diameter. It lies in the great omentum on its way to the spleen. It also has a branch to the pancreas and several small gastric branches that form anastomoses with branches of the left gastric artery.

### 8.1.2 Cranial mesenteric artery

This is the largest visceral branch of the abdominal aorta; it is about 5–10 mm caudal to the coeliac artery and about 5 mm in diameter; it is located at the level of the first or second lumbar vertebrae. Like the coeliac artery it is surrounded by the coeliacomesenteric nerve plexus and numerous lymphatic vessels. It gives rise to several arteries

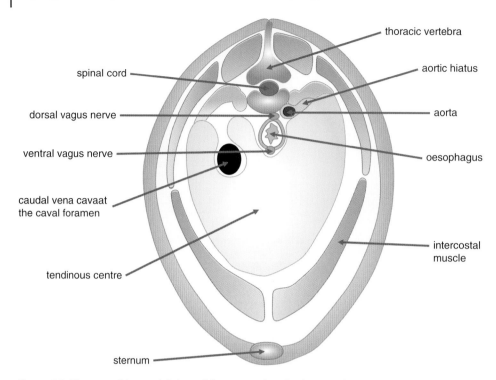

Figure 8.3 Diagram of the cranial view of the mammalian diaphragm. This example shows the azygos vein on the right so therefore must belong to a horse or a carnivore (see Section 9.1.2).

supplying blood to the intestines. Its branches are the **common colic** artery, the **middle colic** artery, the **right colic** artery, the **ileocolic** artery, the **caudal pancreaticoduodenal** artery and the multiple **jejunal** arteries.

The common colic artery is the first of the branches of the cranial mesenteric artery and is about 2 cm from the aorta. It gives rise to several branches, e.g. middle colic and right colic arteries, before becoming the ileocecocolic artery. There are several arterial branches of these vessels supplying the viscera and named according to the intestines and omenta that are supplied. In addition, there are many anastomoses.

### 8.1.3  Phrenicoabdominal arteries

These are paired parietal branches that supply the adrenal glands via the suprarenal arteries, the diaphragm via the **caudal phrenic** artery and the abdominal wall via the **cranial abdominal** artery. It does seem likely that these two arteries are only found in carnivores. *NAV* is not clear on their existence in other species.

### 8.1.4  Renal arteries

These are paired arteries supplying the kidneys. The right one is about 2 cm cranial to the left, conforming with the positioning of the kidneys, and about 3–4 mm in diameter. The renal arteries each supply at least two small branches to the caudal pole of the adjacent adrenal gland. The renal arteries often divide into several interlobar arteries before reaching the kidney hilus. See Chapter 12 for further discussion of the arterial supply to the kidneys.

### 8.1.5 Lumbar segmental arteries

The seven paired lumbar arteries are parietal branches of the aorta. Five of the arteries are branches of the abdominal aorta, and the cranial two are branches of the thoracic aorta. Each artery divides into a dorsal and a spinal branch. The dorsal branches supply the epaxial muscles and cutaneous tissues. The spinal branches enter the spinal canal with the spinal nerves.

### 8.1.6 Gonadal arteries

The paired **ovarian** arteries arise from the aorta about halfway between the renal and **external iliac** arteries. They follow a tortuous course through the broad ligaments to the ovaries. Branches supply the ovary, the ovarian bursa, the uterine cornu and the uterine tube. The branch to the uterine cornu anastomoses with the **uterine** artery, a branch of the **internal iliac** artery.

The **testicular** artery leaves the aorta at the corresponding level of the ovarian artery. Together with the testicular vein the artery enters the **mesorchium** (see Section 16.4 and Figure 16.2. This is the only artery supplying the testis and epididymis.

### 8.1.7 Caudal mesenteric artery

Arising as a single artery on the ventral aspect of the aorta at the level of the fifth lumbar vertebra in the dog (fourth lumbar vertebra in the horse), this artery reaches the distal extremity of the descending colon, where it bifurcates into the **caudal rectal** and **left colic** arteries; the latter anastomoses with the right colic artery.

The left colic artery lies within the mesocolon accompanying the descending colon until there is an anastomosis between the left colic and middle colic arteries.

### 8.1.8 Deep circumflex iliac arteries

These small paired arteries arise from the aorta about 1 cm cranial to the origin of the external iliac arteries. They supply the adjacent body wall via deep and superficial branches.

### 8.1.9 External iliac arteries

The external iliac artery is the largest parietal branch of the abdominal aorta. It is the principal artery to the hindlimb and divides into **femoral** and **deep femoral** branches before leaving the trunk to enter the hindlimb.

### 8.1.10 Internal iliac arteries

The aorta terminates just caudal to the origin of the external iliac arteries as a bifurcation into the pair of internal iliac arteries and the single median sacral artery.

The **umbilical** artery arises from the internal iliac near its origin and has different functions in the female depending on the presence of pregnancy. It is only functional during pregnancy when it carries blood from the aorta to the placenta. In the absence of pregnancy its lumen is obliterated, and it becomes the lateral umbilical ligament.

The internal iliac artery gives rise to visceral and parietal divisions. The **urogenital** and **internal pudendal** arteries belong to the visceral division. The parietal division includes the iliolumbar and the gluteal arteries.

In the male the **artery of the penis** terminates the internal pudendal artery and gives origin to the **artery of the bulb of the penis, the deep artery of the penis** and the **dorsal artery of the penis.**

In the female the cranial branch of the urogenital artery is the **uterine artery**. This artery varies in size depending on the physiological state of the reproductive tract. It courses through the broad ligament and sends small branches to the round ligament, the ovarian bursa and ovary. The **artery of the clitoris** is the terminus of the visceral internal pudendal artery.

## 8.2   Species Variations

The description of the abdominal and pelvic arteries in this chapter is based on the dog. There are very close similarities between the domestic mammals, any differences being due to the variations in gross anatomy. For example, the contrast between the ruminant and equine abdominal viscera inevitably leads to variation in vascularity.

There are few circumstances in which the abdominal arteries are directly involved in clinical situations. Neoplastic lesions of the abdominal and pelvic organs may cause haemorrhage, and mechanical injuries of the gastrointestinal and reproductive viscera may damage blood vessels. Large redworms (*Strongylus vulgaris*) migrate within equine blood vessels, especially the cranial mesenteric artery, causing haemorrhage. However, the attentive use of anthelmintic preparations has considerably reduced the occurrence of these parasites.

# 9

# Veins of the Abdomen and Pelvis (Figure 9.1)

The **caudal vena cava** is the main drainage channel for venous blood from the abdomen and pelvis to the heart. There are a number of tributaries arising from the abdominal body wall and from the kidneys and gonads. The **portal system** conveys venous blood from the stomach, intestines, pancreas and spleen to the liver from which the blood enters the **caudal vena cava** for passage to the heart.

## 9.1 Tributaries of the Caudal Vena Cava

The paired **internal iliac veins** join the **external iliac veins**, and the two **common iliac veins** converge at the level of the seventh lumbar vertebra in carnivores (L6 in the horse and ruminants, L6/L7 in the pig). The **caudal vena cava** then continues cranially in the roof of the abdomen and on the right side of the aorta. When the vena cava reaches the liver, it inclines ventrally before passing through the diaphragm at the **caval foramen** (see Figure 8.3).

### 9.1.1 Deep circumflex iliac veins

These paired veins join the vena cava at the level of the junction of the common iliac veins. They correspond to the arteries of the same name.

### 9.1.2 Lumbar veins

Seven pairs of **lumbar veins** correspond to the lumbar segmental arteries. The first two lumbar veins (i.e. the most caudal) are tributaries of the **azygos vein**. In the horse and carnivores it is the right azygos vein that becomes functional. In the ox, sheep and pig it is the left azygos vein that persists. The right azygos vein (formerly called the **hemiazygos vein**) drains into the final part of the **cranial vena cava** (or sometimes the right atrium of the heart). The left azygos vein enters the **right atrium** at the coronary sinus, the terminus of the great coronary vein. The azygos vein drains most of the blood from the vertebral venous sinuses.

*King's Applied Anatomy of the Abdomen and Pelvis of Domestic Mammals*, First Edition. Geoff Skerritt.
© 2022 John Wiley & Sons Ltd. Published 2022 by John Wiley & Sons Ltd.
Companion website: www.wiley.com/go/skerritt/abdomen

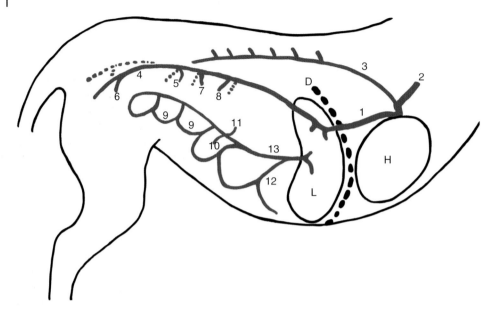

Figure 9.1 Diagram of the abdominal veins of the dog. Note that the right veins only are labelled where the veins are paired. D = diaphragm; L = liver; H = heart. 1 = caudal vena cava; 2 = cranial vena cava; 3 = right azygos; 4 = external iliac; 5 = right deep circumflex; 6 = right internal iliac; 7 = right testicular/ovarian; 8 = right renal; 9 = jejunal; 10 = caudal mesenteric; 11 = splenic; 12 = gastroduodenal; 13 = portal

### 9.1.3   The gonadal veins

The **testicular veins** receive blood from the testis and epididymis. They become coiled, tortuous and intertwined with the artery, lymphatics and nerves; this arrangement is called the **pampiniform plexus** (see Sections 16.4 and 16.5). The right testicular vein enters the caudal vena cava just caudal to the right renal vein. The **left testicular vein** or the **left ovarian vein** enters the left renal vein.

The **right ovarian vein** is at the same location as the male vessel, but it is less tortuous than its homologue. It receives several tributaries from the ovary and adjacent tissues. The uterine arterial tributary forms an anastomosis with the uterine vein (a tributary of the external iliac vein) within the broad ligament.

### 9.1.4   Renal veins

The paired renal veins are quite short, and they are 6–8 mm in diameter. The left renal vein receives the left testicular vein in the male and the left ovarian vein in the female.

### 9.1.5   Phrenicoabdominal veins

These paired veins enter the vena cava just cranial to the renal veins. They cross the ventral surface in a groove on the ventral surface of the corresponding adrenal gland (suprarenal gland, *NAV*). They receive blood from the diaphragm and the body wall.

### 9.1.6   Hepatic veins

There are at least 20 tributaries of various sizes draining the liver lobes to the vena cava before it passes through the diaphragm.

### 9.1.7   Phrenic veins

These paired veins drain the diaphragm and enter the vena cava just as it passes through the diaphragm.

## 9.2   The Hepatic Portal Vein

This is the major route of venous drainage from the gastrointestinal organs, the pancreas, the spleen and the rectum. It arises from a capillary bed in the mesojejunum and terminates in the hepatic capillary bed. There are three main tributaries corresponding to the three arteries that supply the gastrointestinal organs:

- Gastrosplenic tributary draining the intra-abdominal oesophagus, the stomach, early duodenum, pancreas and the spleen. It is about 5 mm in diameter.
- Cranial mesenteric vein draining the small intestine via the jejunal veins that accompany the corresponding arteries.
- Caudal mesenteric vein originating as the cranial rectal vein, which then gathers several tributaries, namely the ileocaecocolic, common colic, left and right colic veins.

The distal rectum and anus are drained via the paired internal iliac veins, which then drain to the caudal vena cava via the common iliac veins.

The hepatic portal vein enters the liver at the porta together with hepatic arteries, nerves and the bile duct; this gateway to the liver is termed the hilus (see Section 7.2).

## 9.3   The Mammary Glands

These modified sweat glands are discussed in this chapter because they are highly vascular and the distribution of their veins is more extensive than their arteries. Collectively called mammae, their function is to provide a source of nutrients for the newborn. They are rudimentary in the male, but in the female their activity is related to pregnancy and a period of lactation following the birth of progeny. In both sexes the mammary glands are typically arranged in pairs either side of the midline on the ventral aspect of the abdomen and/or pelvis; their numbers vary with the species and individual. Following ovulation there is some swelling of the glands. If pregnancy occurs there is marked hyperplasia of the glandular tissue.

A mammary gland consists of glandular tissue arranged in lobules and consisting of secretory epithelial cells arranged in spherical alveoli. The secretion (milk) collects in the lumen of an alveolus and then enters a duct system that conducts it to a teat, or nipple, on the surface of the mammary gland. The mammary secretions correspond to gestation so that they are timed to commence with parturition. The first secretions are of colostrum, a milk precursor containing antibodies, immunoglobulins and growth factors. It is very important that the newborn animal receives this protective cocktail of antibodies. This is particularly important in farm animals because the epitheliochorial placenta is a barrier to the passage of antibodies from maternal to foetal blood circulation.

The number of ducts opening on a teat varies by species and individual. The gland sinus receives secretion, which then drains into a teat sinus and then via the teat canal to a teat orifice.

The mammary glands are extremely vascular. In the bitch they receive their blood supply from the internal thoracic artery, a branch of the subclavian artery in the thorax and the pudendoepigastric artery, a branch of the external iliac artery. These arteries are further distributed in the ventral body wall as the cranial and caudal epigastric arteries. The mammary glands are drained by the cranial and caudal superficial epigastric veins. In the bitch the two cranial mammary glands also drain directly into the internal thoracic vein.

### 9.3.1 Species variations

**Horse:** There are only two mammary glands in the mare. They are located at the junction between the abdomen and pelvis; they are relatively small and are concealed from view by the thighs. Each gland has a single teat that is small except when lactating. The secretory tissues of the two glands are combined and difficult to separate.

**Ox:** There are four mammary glands in the cow. Commonly called the udder, the four glands, each with a teat, are combined as a single unit, but with a midline groove separating left from right. The udder of a lactating dairy cow can weigh at least 50 kg. Accessory teats can be present, each with glandular tissue but often interfering with milking. The cranial and caudal glands on the same side are usually combined. The skin of the udder is thin and mobile with a covering of fine hair.

Following ovulation there is some swelling of the glands. If pregnancy occurs there is marked hyperplasia of the glandular tissue.

The number of ducts opening on a teat varies by species and individual. The gland sinus receives secretion, which then drains into a teat sinus and then via the teat canal to a teat orifice. The skin of the udder is thin and mobile with a covering of fine hair.

The symphyseal tendon originates from the pelvic symphysis and provides a common origin for the gracilis and adductor muscles as well as the suspensory apparatus of the udder. The collagenous lateral laminae of the suspensory apparatus attach to the right and left aspects of the udder. The cranial parts of the lateral laminae originate from the yellow elastic tunic on the lateral side of the superficial inguinal ring (see Section 1.3.2).

The main arterial supply to the udder is provided by the external pudendal artery, a branch of the deep femoral artery. On entry to the udder the artery forms a sigmoid flexure to allow extension when the udder is full of milk. This artery then divides into a large cranial mammary artery and a small caudal mammary artery. There are many anastomoses between the many branches entwined with the lactiferous sinuses. The arrangement of the venous drainage is more complex. There is a venous ring at the base of the udder that collects the blood from the glands; it then leaves the ring via a large subcutaneous abdominal vein to enter the internal thoracic vein followed by the cranial vena cava. Many large superficial lymphatic channels conduct lymph to the mammary lymph nodes.

**Sheep:** The udder of the sheep and goat is located in the inguinal region and comprises two mammary glands. There is variation in the shape of the teats and the amount of hair cover. With regard to the topography and vascularity the udder is similar to that of the cow.

**Pig:** The sow usually has seven or eight mammary glands distributed over the ventral aspect of the thoracic, abdominal and inguinal body wall. In other respects the mammary glands of the pig are similar to those of the ruminants.

**Dog and cat:** The number of mammary glands in the bitch varies from 8 to 12, but there is commonly a reduced number in the smaller breeds. In the cat there are six to eight glands. The secretory tissue is prominent only during pregnancy, lactation, pseudopregnancy and for a period about 45 days while the bitch or queen is nursing. The structure of the mammary glands is basically the same as in the other domestic mammals. The highly vascular mammary glands derive their vascularity from the epigastric arteries, branches of the internal thoracic arteries. There is a rich network of lymphatic vessels and lymph nodes associated with the mammary tissues.

Clinical disease of the mammary glands is common in the bitch, especially neoplasia and mastitis. Malignant neoplasia usually requires radical excision and even so involvement of the lymphatic tissues conveys a poor prognosis.

# 10

# Lymphatics and the Spleen

## 10.1 The Lymphatic System (Figure 10.1)

The mammalian body has a second system of organs and channels similar to the blood circulatory system; it is called the lymphatic system. The system carries an aqueous solution (lymph) containing lymphocytes that protect the body from infection. The lymphocytes are generated in the bone marrow and are found in concentration in the spleen, thymus and tonsils as well as in numerous bean-like nodules called **lymph nodes** that act as filters of the lymph and centres of production of lymphocytes. Lymph nodes consist of a capsule surrounding a cortex and medulla. There are very many lymph nodes throughout the body; some of the lymph nodes are palpable (e.g. in the axilla, behind the stifle and ventral to the mandible). If large numbers of bacteria are filtered by a lymph node, it becomes enlarged and, depending on the location, palpable and the swelling visible. Lymph nodes are located along the abdominal aorta, adjacent to the kidneys and cranial to the external iliac arteries. There are also groups of lymph nodes corresponding to the territories of the three major arteries, viz., coeliac, cranial mesenteric and caudal mesenteric. In the pelvic region there are hypogastric nodes, deep and superficial inguinal nodes draining the reproductive organs and the mammary glands. Aggregations of lymph nodules are located in the small intestine; they are called Peyer's patches.

Nutrients are available to the body tissues by leakage of fluid from the blood capillaries; a major function is the absorption of dietary fats. This interstitial fluid also collects waste products, bacteria and cellular debris, all of which drain into the lymphatic capillaries. In the small intestine the lymphatic capillaries within the villi are called **lacteals**; the lymph then enters lymphatic channels that are progressively of larger diameter, finally becoming a pair of **lymphatic ducts**. The left lymphatic duct is much larger than that on the right and is called the **thoracic duct**. In man both lymphatic ducts drain into the corresponding **subclavian vein** at its junction with the **internal jugular vein**, thereby returning the lymph to the blood circulation. At its origin the thoracic duct is dilated and receives lymph from the intestinal trunk; this dilated part of the thoracic duct is the **cisterna (or receptaculum) chyli**. The cisterna chyli is located dorsal to the aorta and ventral to the cranial lumbar vertebrae. The intestinal trunk collects lymph from the

*King's Applied Anatomy of the Abdomen and Pelvis of Domestic Mammals*, First Edition. Geoff Skerritt.
© 2022 John Wiley & Sons Ltd. Published 2022 by John Wiley & Sons Ltd.
Companion website: www.wiley.com/go/skerritt/abdomen

stomach, intestines, pancreas, spleen and part of the liver. This is the main drainage route for the transport of fatty acids and fats (**chyle**) from the digestive system.

In the domestic mammals there is considerable variation as regards the route by which lymph is returned to the blood circulation. The thoracic duct passes through the **aortic hiatus** (Figure 8.3) into the mediastinum and then usually empties either into the left jugular vein or the caudal vena cava.

## 10.2   The Spleen

The shape and size of the spleen varies amongst the domestic animals (see Figure 10.1) although its location is reasonably constant. The spleen is a flattened, elongated, dark reddish-brown abdominal organ. The spleen is the largest lymphatic organ and structurally resembles a large lymph node. It is located on the left side in the cranial abdomen, most of it being within the caudal rib cage. The visceral side of the spleen is adjacent to the stomach to which it is attached by the **gastrosplenic ligament**; the parietal face lies against the body wall (Figure 3.1).

The fibrous capsule extends by trabeculae into the parenchyma, which consists of two types of tissue identified as **red pulp** and **white pulp**. Most of the spleen is red pulp and consists of mature blood cells, macrophages, plasma cells and lymphocytes. The white pulp consists of lymphoid tissue in discrete nodules, each surrounding a central arteriole. **T (thymus) cells** are adjacent to the arterioles, and then a marginal sinus separates the T cells from macrophages.

**B lymphocytes** predominate in the nodules where they produce antibodies to coat pathogens and facilitate their removal by scavenger cells; 25% of the body's lymphocytes are stored within the spleen.

The **splenic artery** supplies the splenic sinusoids in the red pulp, which act as a filter, preventing old or damaged red blood cells from entering the bloodstream. Bacteria, fungi, viruses and haemoglobin debris are also discarded and phagocytosed. The red pulp also acts as a reservoir for storing blood and blood components, e.g. phagocytes, platelets, haemoglobin and iron. Blood can be released in emergency and sent to sites of injury to facilitate healing. The spleen is a site for haematopoiesis in foetal and neonate animals. The dog's spleen is able to store one-third of the total amount of red cells. In dogs and cats this enables the release of 10–20% of the body's red cells in an emergency.

Despite the apparent important functions of the spleen, it can be removed without serious consequence.

## 10.3   Species Variations

### 10.3.1   Horse

The spleen lies beneath the last three ribs. Dorsally it is broad but narrows cranially and ventrally. On rectal examination it lies against the body wall and feels smooth with a sharp border. The spleen can contract and release red blood cells in response to strenuous exercise. The nephrosplenic (renosplenic) ligament connects the left kidney to the spleen. The colon can become trapped between this ligament and the spleen, resulting in colic (Figure 10.1).

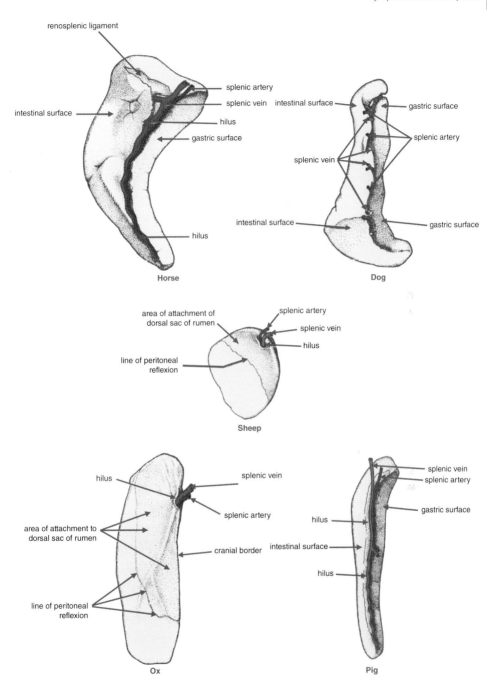

Figure 10.1 Visceral surface of the spleen of the domestic species.

### 10.3.2   Ruminants

The spleen is flat and oblong-shaped. The ventral end of the spleen is in contact with the reticulum in the ox. Nodules of lymphoid tissue, splenic corpuscles, are prominent on the cut surface of the spleen. The spleen of the sheep is relatively smaller than that of the ox.

### 10.3.3   Pig

The spleen is long and strap-like, lying under the last three ribs. It is very similar to the spleen of ox, complete with splenic corpuscles.

### 10.3.4   Carnivore

The spleen is long and dumbbell-shaped, wider ventrally. The location of the spleen depends on the size of the stomach. It is attached to the greater curvature of the stomach by the gastrosplenic ligament.

### 10.3.5   Whale

Uniquely there are up to 14 separate small spleens in these mammals.

## 10.4   Clinical Conditions Affecting the Lymphatic System

- **Splenomegaly** is enlargement of the spleen and can be either localised or generalised. Localised splenomegaly can be an abscess, neoplasia, hyperplasia or a haematoma. Generalised splenomegaly may be neoplastic, e.g. leukaemia; inflammatory, e.g. hepatitis; hyperplastic, e.g. bacterial endocarditis; or congestive, e.g. splenic torsion.
- **Lymphosarcoma** (lymphoma) is common in dogs and cats and can involve the liver, lymph nodes, bone marrow, the spleen and commonly in the intestine. Cats that are positive for leukaemia (feline leukaemia virus [FeLV]) are more likely to develop lymphosarcoma. Certain dog breeds are more susceptible to lymphosarcoma, e.g. Boxers, Golden Retrievers and Basset Hounds. The clinical signs include enlargement of lymph nodes, loss of appetite, loss of weight, vomiting, diarrhoea and lethargy. Lymphosarcoma can affect any organ containing lymphocytes, e.g. kidneys, spinal cord and skin. The disease results in the proliferation of malignant lymphocytes.

  A vaccine against FeLV is available for cats. Chemotherapy is the best treatment but the disease is often fatal.
- **Lymphadenopathy** is the term generally used to describe disease affecting the lymph nodes. Reactive hyperplasia of lymph nodes is the enlargement of lymph nodes in response to the pathology of the tissues filtered by those lymph nodes. There are many substances that are carried to the lymph nodes; some are harmless and are simply phagocytosed, while others cause an immune reaction resulting in swelling of the affected lymph nodes. Examples of causative agents are bacteria, viruses, chemicals and neoplastic cells.

- **Feline leukaemia virus** only affects cats. It is caused by a transmissible retrovirus and is invariably fatal. The clinical signs are anaemia, weight loss, fatigue, oral disease and enlargement of lymph nodes. The disease is highly contagious and is transmitted in saliva, urine, faeces and nasal secretions. An effective vaccine is available and is recommended.
- **Haemangiosarcoma in dogs.** This serious condition is invariably fatal unless emergency surgery is carried out. One survey concluded that one in five Golden Retrievers will suffer this neoplastic disease. It is the endothelial cells lining the blood vessels of the spleen that become neoplastic. Apart from a swollen abdomen and anaemia there are few clinical signs until the spleen ruptures. A weak pulse, pale mucous membranes, rapid heart rate and panting may be apparent. Haemangiomas can occur elsewhere, e.g. liver or skin, but are most frequent in the spleen. Emergency surgery, usually removal of the spleen and a blood transfusion followed by chemotherapy, gives the best chance of survival.

# 11

# The Nerves of the Abdomen and Pelvis

There are five functional divisions of the nervous system. Formerly the basis of classification was the division into somatic and autonomic (visceral) systems with sensory (afferent) and motor (efferent) subdivisions. The neurons of one of these divisions are restricted to the head; these belong to the special visceral efferent (SVE) neuronal component (also called branchial efferent). These neurons innervate the muscles developed from the pharyngeal arches and contribute to:

- The trigeminal nerve supplying the chewing muscles
- The facial nerve supplying the facial muscles
- Cranial nerves IX and X–XI supplying pharyngeal and laryngeal muscles.

There are no SVE neurons supplying the organs or tissues of the abdomen and pelvis.

The division between somatic and autonomic components of the nervous system becomes extremely difficult since many bodily functions involve both somatic (e.g. skeletal muscles) and autonomic activity (e.g. adjustments in blood circulation). In summary, motor (efferent) axons innervating skeletal muscle are somatic, whereas axons innervating smooth muscle and glandular tissue are autonomic.

## 11.1 General Somatic Afferent Neurons

The general somatic afferent (GSA) neurons of the abdomen and pelvis have their cell bodies in the **dorsal root ganglia** of the lumbar and sacral segmental spinal nerves. The dorsal root ganglia are located within the vertebral canal at the level of each intervertebral foramen. The dorsal root is joined by the ventral root, and as soon as the nerves leave the vertebral canal they divide into dorsal and ventral branches. Both of these branches contain GSA neurons that originate at a variety of cutaneous receptors responding to touch, pain, pressure and temperature in the wall of the abdomen and pelvis.

## 11.2 General Visceral Afferent Neurons

The receptors of the general visceral afferent (GVA) system are found within the viscera of the body and respond to a variety of stimuli, e.g. stretch and distention of the viscera, chemical and temperature, changes in the environment, and movement of the viscera.

*King's Applied Anatomy of the Abdomen and Pelvis of Domestic Mammals*, First Edition. Geoff Skerritt.
© 2022 John Wiley & Sons Ltd. Published 2022 by John Wiley & Sons Ltd.
Companion website: www.wiley.com/go/skerritt/abdomen

These GVA neurons in the abdomen and pelvis enter the **vagus** (X) nerve and ascend to the nucleus of the solitary tract in the brainstem as well as forming reflex arcs with general visceral efferent (GVE) neurons.

## 11.3 General Somatic Efferent Neurons

The general somatic efferent (GSE) neuron is the lower motor neuron (LMN) of the peripheral nervous system. In the abdomen and pelvis the cell bodies of the GSE neurons are located in the **ventral horn** of the spinal cord. The axons of these neurons leave the spinal cord to enter the lumbar and sacral spinal nerves. The majority of the motor axons are distributed to the striated muscles of the trunk.

## 11.4 General Visceral Efferent Neurons

These motor pathways (GVE) belong to the autonomic system and are divided into the sympathetic and parasympathetic divisions. The sympathetic system is responsible for widespread visceral responses required in emergency, the so-called 'fight or flight response'. The parasympathetic system is responsible for the visceral responses that are required for the maintenance of the body's reserves and tends to act locally. The two systems often act antagonistically, although some organs are innervated by the sympathetic system **only** (e.g. the adrenal medulla, sweat glands and many blood vessels).

The two systems act through different transmitter substances at their effector endings; these are noradrenaline or adrenaline at sympathetic effector endings and acetylcholine at parasympathetic endings.

### 11.4.1 Sympathetic motor pathways (Figures 11.1, 11.2, 11.3, 11.4 and 11.7)

The sympathetic outflow from the central nervous system (CNS) is limited to the thoracic and rostral lumbar segments of the spinal cord; it extends to as far as L1 to L5 depending on species. The cell bodies of these preganglionic sympathetic neurons are located in the **lateral horn** of the spinal cord and represent the entire outflow of sympathetic motor pathways to the whole of the body. Their myelinated axons leave the cord by the ventral root, enter a white ramus communicans and end in one of a chain of **vertebral ganglia** (ganglia of the sympathetic trunk, *NAV*).

The preganglionic neurons form synapses with several postganglionic neurons in the vertebral ganglia. In fact the ratio of pre- to postganglionic neurons is high, about 1:20 or more. The axons of the postganglionic neurons return to the spinal nerves via an unmyelinated grey ramus communicans.

In the abdomen (originating in segments T6–T10 in the cat) the axons of the preganglionic neurons pass straight through the vertebral ganglia and contribute to the **great splanchnic nerve**. The axon ends by entering a **prevertebral ganglion**,

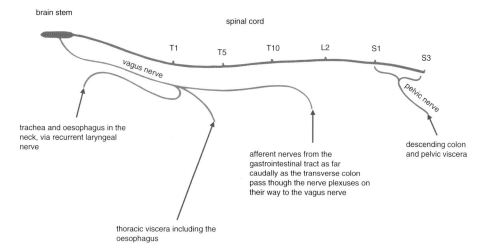

**Figure 11.1** Summary of the afferent pathways from the viscera, excluding pain. The non-pain sensory nerve pathways from the thoracic, abdominal and pelvic viscera travel to the neuraxis in the vagus and pelvic nerves.

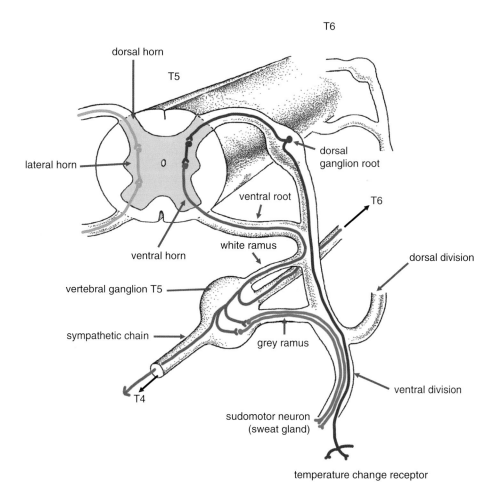

**Figure 11.2** Diagram to show the sympathetic motor pathway of the somatic region of the abdomen. The example shows a receptor sensitive to temperature change, and the effector is a sudomotor neuron.

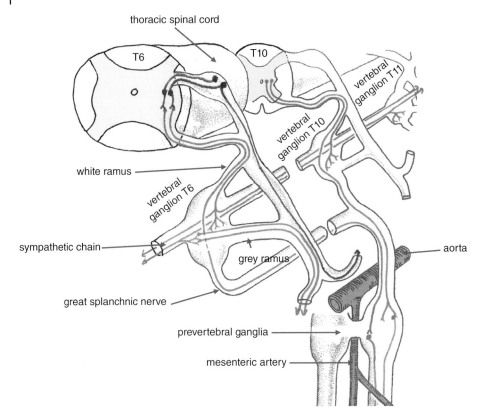

**Figure 11.3** Diagram of the sympathetic motor pathway to the viscera. Refer to Figure 11.2 for the colour code. The preganglionic nerves originating in segments T6–T10 (in the cat) pass through the vertebral ganglia and enter the greater splanchnic nerve. They continue into the coeliacomesenteric plexus to synapse in a prevertebral ganglion with many postganglionic neurons, which are then distributed to target organs.

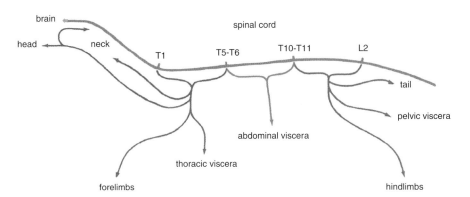

**Figure 11.4** Summary of the motor outflow of the sympathetic system. The diagram is based on the cat, in which a total of 15 segments (T1 to L2 inclusive) contribute to the sympathetic outflow from the neuraxis. These 15 segments can be divided functionally into three groups, each consisting of five segments. These three groups supply particular regions of the body, essentially as shown.

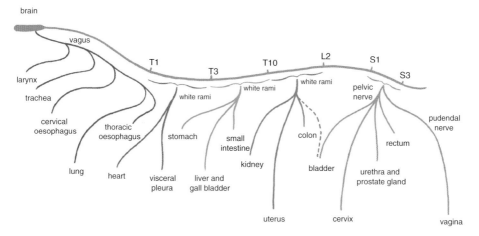

**Figure 11.5** Summary of the pain pathways from the viscera. The great majority of the pain pathways from the viscera are projected to the CNS by axons that travel in sympathetic nerves. Topographically these pain pathways tend to resemble the motor pathways of the sympathetic system (see Figure 11.4). Thus, both the motor pathways and the pain pathways of the thoracic viscera travel mainly in the sympathetic nerves relating to the segments T1–T5; likewise both the motor pathways and the pain pathways to the abdominal viscera travel mainly in the sympathetic nerves relating to the segments T6–T10. However, the pain pathways from the pelvic viscera break with this principle by projecting to the CNS via the pelvic and pudendal nerves rather than via the sympathetic nerves relating to segments T11–L2. The pain pathways from the respiratory tract including the lung form another exception by travelling in the vagus.

where it forms numerous branches that synapse with about 20 postganglionic neurons. Again the ratio of pre- to postganglionic neurons is therefore about 1:20, as in the vertebral ganglia.

The prevertebral ganglia (ganglia of the autonomic plexuses, *NAV*) arise as paired primordia that fuse to varying extents. They lie on the ventral aspect of the dorsal aorta, and the left ganglion tends to fuse with that on the right.

There are a number of prevertebral ganglia in the abdomen. The most important are the coeliac, cranial mesenteric and caudal mesenteric ganglia. The coeliac and cranial mesenteric ganglia become fused in many species to form a composite **coeliacomesenteric ganglion** that supplies postganglionic nerves to the abdominal viscera. These sympathetic nerves travel to their target organs along the arteries, which supply these organs, e.g. the axons supplying the wall of the stomach travel along the branches of the coeliac artery. The **caudal mesenteric ganglion** distributes sympathetic postganglionic axons via the **hypogastric nerves** to the pelvic viscera, e.g. the urogenital organs, rectum, etc.

### 11.4.2 The prevertebral ganglia (Figures 11.1 and 11.2)

The prevertebral ganglia contain postganglionic neurons of three functional types:

- Vasomotor to blood vessels of the gastrointestinal tract
- Motor to the smooth muscle in the wall of the gastrointestinal tract
- Motor to the glands of the of the gastrointestinal tract.

The vasomotor fibres are very numerous and strongly influence the systemic arterial blood pressure by constituting a variable resistance to the output of the left ventricle. For example, if the blood pressure falls because of haemorrhage, a reflex vasoconstriction of the splanchnic circulation occurs.

The sympathetic innervation of the smooth muscle of the gut causes the sphincters to close and the intestine wall to relax. Hence the movement of ingesta is arrested.

Also, in line with a 'fight or flight' response, the sympathetic innervation of the glands of the intestine promotes inhibition.

### 11.4.3 Sympathetic transmitter substances

Preganglionic sympathetic axons release acetylcholine at their endings and are called cholinergic fibres. Many interneurons in the CNS also release acetylcholine at their endings.

Most postganglionic sympathetic axons release adrenaline or noradrenaline at their endings; they are called adrenergic fibres. There are some exceptions, e.g. the sympathetic postganglionic nerves that innervate merocrine sweat glands and sympathetic vasodilator fibres are cholinergic.

The endocrine cells of the **adrenal medulla** are derived embryologically from neural crest tissue and release noradrenaline or adrenaline. The medullary cells are the equivalent of postganglionic cells that are without axons.

### 11.4.4 Pain pathways from the abdominal viscera (Figure 11.5 and 11.6)

Most of the pathways of visceral pain are carried in the sympathetic nerves. The visceral peritoneum and the gastrointestinal tract are insensitive to crushing and cutting, but they are painful when stretched or subject to muscular spasm. These GVA pathways accompany the sympathetic GVE pathways and pass through the white rami on their way to the dorsal root ganglia of segments T5–L2. However, the pain pathways from the pelvic viscera travel in the **pelvic** and **pudendal nerves** via the dorsal root ganglia to the sacral segments of the spinal cord.

### 11.4.5 Parasympathetic motor pathways (Figure 11.7)

In general the function of the parasympathetic motor pathways is to conserve the reserves of the organism. Both the pre- and the postganglionic parasympathetic endings release acetylcholine.

The outflow of parasympathetic preganglionic pathways is restricted to the sacral and cranial regions of the CNS. However, the vagus nerve provides the pathway for the parasympathetic nerve supply to the gastrointestinal organs. The parasympathetic postganglionic neurons are located between the longitudinal and circular muscle layers of the gut and are called the **myenteric**, or **Auerbach's plexus**. There is also some sympathetic input to this plexus and even a sensory component.

The sacral outflow originates from the sacral segments of the spinal cord and is related to the number of sacral vertebrae in each species, e.g. S1, S2 and S3 in the cat and dog, S1–S5 in the horse and ox. The cell bodies of the preganglionic neurons are located at a site that corresponds to the lateral horn of the spinal cord. The axons are combined as the **pelvic nerve** (renamed as the **splanchnic nerve** in *NAV*). Its main

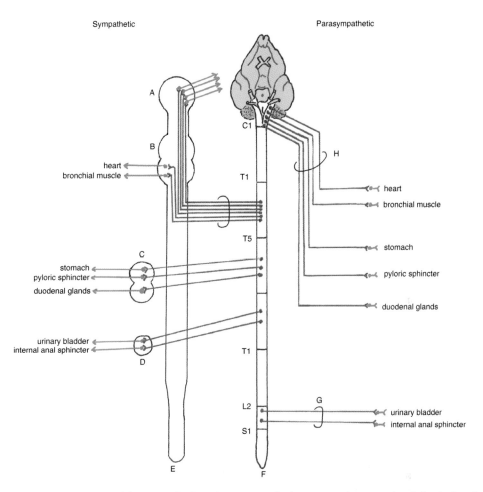

**Figure 11.6** Diagram of the sympathetic and parasympathetic motor pathways to the abdominal and pelvic viscera. A = cranial cervical ganglion; B = stellate ganglion; C = coeliacomesentreic ganglion; D = caudalmesenteric ganglion; E = sympathetic chain; F = spinal cord; G = pelvic nerve; H = vagus nerve; J = great splanchnic nerve.

function is to open smooth muscle sphincters in the pelvic viscera and, at the same time, to contract the muscle in the walls of the bladder and rectum. The pelvic nerve also contains parasympathetic vasodilator nerve fibres to the erectile tissue of the penis.

Both the anus and bladder also have external sphincters of striated muscle that are innervated by GSE fibres. The external anal sphincter is innervated by the **pudendal nerve**.

## 11.5 Clinical Conditions

Amongst the domestic animals there are two examples of clinical conditions that primarily affect the autonomic nervous system; they are called **dysautonomias**. In the horse the disease became known as grass sickness due to the apparent association with

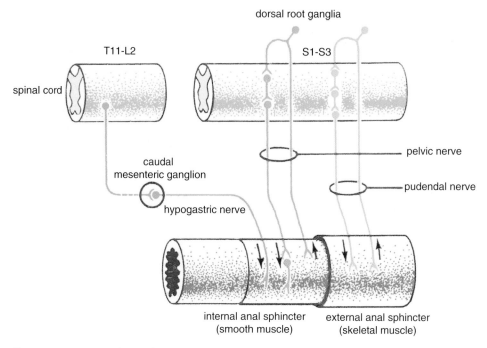

**Figure 11.7** Diagram of the reflexive innervation of the anal sphincters of the dog. The internal sphincter consists of smooth muscle. The external sphincter is skeletal muscle.

grazing on lush grass in Spring or Autumn. It is a serious disease with a high mortality rate. The clinical signs include abdominal pain and distension, salivation, inappetance and tachycardia.

Dysautonomia in cats, also known as Key-Gaskell syndrome, is characterised by widespread degeneration of both pre- and postganglionic neurons of the sympathetic and parasympathetic systems. The clinical signs in affected cats include anorexia, constipation, abdominal distension, pupillary dilatation, reduced tear secretion, protrusion of the third eyelid, atony of the urinary bladder, regulation of smooth muscle and secretion of glands. Dysautonomia has recently been reported in a number of species including young dogs but occurs primarily in cats.

In the domestic animals the principal clinical situation that involves the nerves of the abdominal/pelvic organs belongs to the lumbosacral spinal cord. In addition, the species most likely to suffer such a such a disorder are the dog and cat. From the T11 to the S1 vertebrae there is a possibility of a protrusion of an intervertebral disc. **Chondrodystrophoid** dog breeds (e.g. Dachshund, Basset Hound and Corgi) are particularly prone to this condition because their discs undergo premature degeneration. The clinical signs of a disc protrusion usually involve disturbance of the GSA and GSE pathways especially supplying the hindlimbs. It is perhaps surprising that the sympathetic pathways do not show more evidence of their inevitable involvement.

**Vagus indigestion** in ruminants was originally thought to be the result of lesions actually involving the vagus nerve. However, this chronic ruminoreticular distention is now established not to involve the vagus nerve directly. Any cause of ruminoreticular distention can develop the clinical signs of vagal indigestion although actual damage of the vagus nerve is rarely present.

## 11.6 Regional Anaesthesia

There are a number of regional anaesthetic techniques that enable abdominal surgery with the patient standing. These procedures are almost exclusively reserved for ruminants and have the advantage that the patient remains standing so that there is much less danger of regurgitation.

### 11.6.1 Paravertebral anaesthesia

This technique involves the injection of a local anaesthetic alongside the dorsal and ventral rami of the spinal nerves at T13, L1 and L2 as they emerge from the intervertebral foramina. The technique produces analgesia of the body wall including the parietal peritoneum. The patient remains standing and fully conscious. The GSA neurons that have touch and pain receptors in the body wall are anaesthetised in the localised area. The anaesthetised ventral rami (T13, L1, L2) contain GSE neurons that innervate the striated muscle in the localised region of the body wall. The parasympathetic system does not have any neurons in the thoracolumbar spinal nerves. The sympathetic system does have preganglionic motor neurons within the ventral roots of the thoracolumbar spinal cord. However, the ratio of pre- to postganglionic sympathetic neurons is about 1:20 so that the system is capable of a widespread response or a compensation for the anaesthetised neurons. The result is that, whereas the GSA and GSE neurons are effectively anaesthetised, there are plenty of sympathetic GVA neurons to maintain function.

### 11.6.2 Pudendal nerve block

This procedure is used to produce anaesthesia of the penis and prepuce of the bull. The main trunk of the pudendal nerve divides into two terminal branches:

1) The dorsal nerve of the penis supplying GSE fibres to the retractor penis muscle and GSA fibres providing sensory innervation to the free end of the penis.
2) The superficial perineal nerve, which divides into a preputial branch providing sensation (GSA) to the preputial membrane and a scrotal branch supplying cutaneous sensation (GSA) to the scrotum.

In addition, there is a pudendal branch of the ischiatic nerve that originates from spinal segments L6, S1 and S2 and that can also be anaesthetised. The procedure involves rectal palpation and anaesthesia of the pudendal nerve in the ischiatic foramen.

Epidural anaesthesia is now preferred to pudendal nerve block.

# 12

# The Kidneys (Figures 12.1 and 12.2)

## 12.1 Nitrogenous Excretion

The kidneys are paired bean-shaped organs found in vertebrates. Their shape, size and location vary with species as described below, but in mammals they are found either side of the major vascular vessels, the aorta and caudal vena cava, in the roof of the abdomen. The kidneys are covered by parietal peritoneum and so are outside the peritoneal cavity. The kidneys receive blood via the renal arteries, short, large-diameter branches of the dorsal aorta. The renal veins drain blood directly to the caudal vena cava. The function of the kidneys is to filter the blood and extract urine, which is passed through the **ureters** to the urinary bladder. The functional unit of a kidney is the **nephron**.

There is some confusion in regard to the terminology used to name the components of the nephron. The nomenclature has been updated (*NAV*), and the most recent terms are used here. Each nephron includes a bundle of capillaries through which blood passes from afferent to efferent arterioles. This vascular knot is called a **glomerulus** and is surrounded by a **Bowman's capsule**, the name retained for the double-layered hemisphere that is the blind-ending of the proximal convoluted tubule. The whole unit of glomerulus and Bowman's capsule is termed a **renal corpuscle**.

Further confusion surrounds the naming of some of the gross anatomical components of the kidney. The **renal pelvis** is the compartment that drains directly into the ureter. There is no boundary between the renal pelvis and the **major calyx**, so that they are effectively the same. Urine passes from the Bowman's capsule into the **proximal convoluted tubule**, which is separated from the **distal convoluted tubule** by an elongated mid-section called the **hairpin loop**. This extension, popularly called the **loop of Henlé**, enters the kidney medulla before returning to the cortex and becoming the distal convoluted tubule. Each **collecting tubule** receives many distal convoluted tubules before becoming a **papillary duct** that drains urine into a **minor calyx** and then into the renal pelvis.

The loop of Henlé is the site of resorption of water and electrolytes. In large dogs up to 2000 litres of blood pass through the kidneys daily, and 200–300 litres are filtered by the glomeruli daily. Following reabsorption by the loops of Henlé, only 1–2 litres of

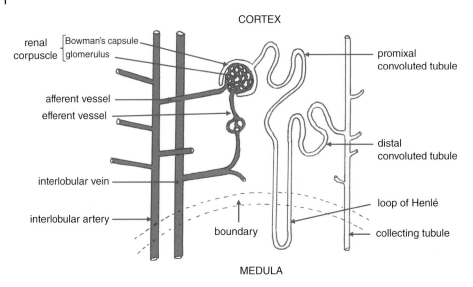

Figure 12.1 Diagram of a nephron showing a filtration arrangement unit for the production of urine.

urine pass through the ureters to the urinary bladder prior to urination. In addition to the voidance of water, certain electrolytes (sodium, potassium, chloride, sulphate and nitrogen compounds such as urea and uric acid) are also excreted.

## 12.2   Gross Anatomy of the Kidneys

The kidneys in all the mammalian species are located retroperitoneally and essentially in a sublumbar position but may extend beneath the last ribs. The right kidney is slightly more cranial than the left and usually fixed into a depression in the liver; the left kidney is more mobile and pendulous. The sublumbar fascia surrounding the kidneys are often well-filled with fat.

Each kidney has an indentation on its medial aspect; this is the **renal sinus** and is the location for the renal vessels and nerves as they enter the kidney at the **renal hilus**. This is also the exit of the **ureter** from its dilated origin, the **renal pelvis**. The kidney is enclosed in a fibrous capsule that protects the inner parenchyma.

The renal parenchyma is divided into an inner medulla and an outer cortex. The cortex contains mainly the renal corpuscles and the convoluted portions of the tubules. The striated appearance of the medulla is due to the presence of very many collecting ducts. The medulla is divided into six to eight **renal pyramids** in the dog; these are cone-shaped with the widest dimension adjacent to the cortex and the apex, or **renal papilla**, directed towards the renal pelvis. At the corticomedullary junction the arcuate arteries are located curving over the bases of the pyramids to give origin to the interlobar arteries.

## 12.3    Species Variations (Figure 12.2)

### 12.3.1    Horse

The kidneys of the horse are not 'kidney-shaped' but are rather 'heart-shaped'. The right kidney is compressed in a craniocaudal direction and is shorter than in the lateromedial dimension. There is little or no external evidence of lobation. The renal pelvis is quite small, comprising only a centrally located collecting cavity. The **renal crest** is small, consisting only of the centrally located renal papillae. The papillary ducts at the extremities drain into one of two large collecting ducts called the terminal recesses, an arrangement found only in the horse.

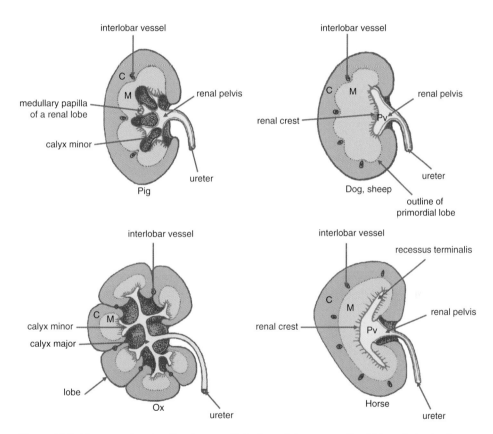

Figure 12.2  Diagrams showing the degree of lobation of the mammalian kidney. Lobation is most marked in the largest mammals and in aquatic animals. C = cortex; M = medulla; shaded areas = renal sinuses occupied by fat and blood vessels. Pig: Lobes present but not visible externally. Several papillae drain into short calyces minores, which empty into two calyces majores. Dog and sheep: Single renal papilla elongated into a renal crest. Blood vessels show lobation. Ox: Lobes present and visible externally as well as internally. Each lobe has a papilla draining into a calyx minor, which empties into one or other of the two calyces majores. No renal pelvis. Horse: Lobation shown only by the blood vessels. The renal crest and the two recessi terminalis receive papillary ducts.

### 12.3.2  Ox

The right kidney of the ox is in contact with the caudate lobe of the liver. Both kidneys are surrounded by a large amount of fat termed the adipose capsule. The lobation of the embryonic kidney is retained in the ox, and there are about 20 lobes grossly visible in each kidney. Each lobe consists of a cortical bulge covering a medullary pyramid. The papillary ducts open into a common chamber called a renal pelvis that, in turn, opens into either the cranial or caudal branch of the ureter.

In adult ruminants the rumen causes the left kidney to be displaced to the right of the midline and to rotate so that the medial side faces dorsally.

### 12.3.3  Sheep

The kidneys of the sheep show no external sign of lobation so that the kidneys of this species are like those of the dog rather than the ox. The renal papillae are in a row called the renal crest that is surrounded by the renal pelvis.

### 12.3.4  Pig

Unlike the other domestic animals, the right kidney is not in contact with the liver. There is no external sign of lobation. Each renal papilla is surrounded by a minor calyx that opens into the renal pelvis or one of two major calyces at the extremities.

### 12.3.5  Dog/cat

In these species the anatomy of the kidneys is as described above in Sections 12.1 and 12.2. There is no external lobation, and the kidneys are bean-shaped and usually embedded in fat. The left kidney lies ventrally to the sublumbar muscles at the level of the second to fourth lumbar vertebrae; the right kidney lies adjacent to the first to third lumbar vertebrae and in a recess of the liver.

In most breeds the left kidney is palpable depending on the obesity of the individual. In the cat there are prominent capsular veins radiating from the hilus.

## 12.4   Clinical Conditions of the Kidneys of the Domestic Mammals

Renal disease is not common in the domestic mammals except in the dog and cat. In **horses** acute renal failure can be a complication of a number of clinical situations, e.g. colic, diarrhoea, dehydration and haemorrhage; with appropriate treatment affected horses usually recover. However, chronic renal failure carries a poor prognosis.

Pyelonephritis in **cattle** is probably more common than realised; it is due to infection with *Corynebacterium renale*. The disease can be either acute or chronic and in both cases results in discoloured urine containing blood and tissue debris. There is usually a response to antibiotic therapy.

Renal infections and congenital malformations do occur in **sheep**. Pulpy kidney disease is really an enterotoxaemia with renal involvement. It is caused by the toxin of

*Clostridium perfringens* Type D but is now controlled by vaccination; the toxin rapidly destroys the renal tubules.

There are several bacteria that can cause pyelonephritis in the **pig**; they are *Actinobaculum suis* (most common), *Staphylococcus hyicus* (greasy pig disease), *Streptococcus* and *Erysipelothrix* (erysipelas).

The incidence of renal disease is highest in **dogs and cats** amongst the domestic mammals. There are many potential causes of nephritis, but the most common is infection with the *Leptospira* bacterium. However, there is an effective vaccine that is best administered annually. There are certain substances which, when ingested, result in serious renal toxicity, e.g. grapes in dogs and lily flowers in cats.

## 12.5    Urinary Bladder and Urethra

The urinary bladder is a hollow, muscular organ that varies in size and position depending on the volume of its contents. In the horse and ox the bladder lies within the pelvic cavity, but in the dog and cat it extends into the abdomen. The wall of the bladder comprises an inner transitional epithelium, three muscle layers and an outer serosa that is actually peritoneum. In the horse and ox the bladder is retroperitoneal, but as it fills with urine it becomes intraperitoneal.

Three vestiges of embryonic structures are visible in the outer wall of the bladder. These are the paired **lateral vesical folds**, originally the **umbilical arteries**, and the median vesicle fold, originally the **urachus**. The lateral vesicle folds become the **round ligaments** of the bladder

The **paired ureteric openings** are located near the neck of the bladder and form a triangle with the exit of the urethra; the arrangement is called the **trigone**.

The urethra of the female lies ventral to the reproductive tract and opens at the junction of the vagina and vestibule. The urethra is lined by a mucous membrane, and its wall comprises circular and longitudinal smooth muscle. The urethra of the mare is short and that of the cow opens in association with a **suburethral diverticulum**. In the bitch the urethra opens on a hillock that can be a problem when inserting a catheter.

The urethra of the male consists of three sections. The first of these passes through the prostate gland, where it receives the paired **deferent ducts**. The middle section is the membranous portion and the distal section is the cavernous (penile) portion.

## 12.6    Adrenal Gland

The pair of adrenal glands are located close to the kidneys on either side. Each gland lies cranially and medially to the corresponding kidney. When sectioned the adrenal gland can be seen to comprise an obvious cortex and medulla. The cortex comprises three zones. The outer zone is the **zona glomerulosa**, the middle zone is the **zona fasciculata** and the inner zone is the **zona reticularis**. The cortex produces steroid hormones – mineralocorticoids (e.g. aldosterone), glucocorticoids (cortisol and cortisone) and androgens.

The functions of the cortical hormones are as follows:

- **Mineralocorticoids:** regulation of blood pressure and concentration of electrolytes
- **Glucocorticoids:** regulation of metabolism and suppression of the immune system
- **Androgens:** production of steroids that are turned into sex hormones in the gonads.

The **chromaffin cells** of the adrenal medulla produce the catecholamines adrenaline and noradrenaline. The adrenal medulla is innervated by sympathetic preganglionic neurones and releases the hormones into the bloodstream (see Section 11.4.3).

### 12.6.1   The blood supply of the adrenal gland

The adrenal gland receives a rich blood supply via the **suprarenal arteries**. These arteries are branches of the phrenicoabdominal (see Section 8.1.3), aortic and renal arteries. In addition, variable arteries arising from the cranial mesenteric and coeliac arteries may be present.

# 13

# The Ovaries and Ovarian Bursae

## 13.1    The Ovary (Figures 13.1 and 13.2)

The ovaries are the paired female **gonads**, homologous to the testes of the male. They include the **ovarian follicles**, each comprising a spherical aggregation of hormone-secreting cells together with a single ovum. The ova are the female germ cells that undergo maturation in the ovaries and are finally released at ovulation. This process begins with a phase of enlargement forming the **primary oocytes**. The first of the two reduction divisions occurs before ovulation, forming the **secondary oocyte** and a **first polar body**. The second reduction division occurs after ovulation, in the uterine tube, and is triggered by the penetration of a spermatozoon; the **ovum** and **second polar body** result. Fertilisation occurs when the male and female pronuclei fuse, forming the **zygote**. The ovary is also an endocrine organ. In all mammals the ovaries are situated in the abdominal cavity, either in the sublumbar region as in the horse and dog or near the pelvic inlet as in the ruminants.

In mammalian females the activity of the ovaries and, to a certain extent the reproductive tract, is controlled by endocrine release; this regular activity is termed the **oestrous cycle**. In human females and in other primates the changes in the reproductive tract are characterised by limited haemorrhage due to shedding of the endometrium, and this activity is called the **menstrual cycle**. However, all mammals lose some endometrium and blood if the ova are not fertilized, but it is not usually a significant amount and, in any case, it is not always a monthly event as implied by the term menstrual (from the Latin *mensis*, meaning month). In non-primates any bleeding is more likely to originate from ovulation and the development of a **corpus haemorrhagicum**. This is followed by the development of a **corpus luteum** (from the Latin meaning 'yellow body') This is a temporary endocrine structure comprising theca cells that produce mainly **progesterone** and **oestradiol**. **Luteinising hormone** (LH) and **follicle-stimulating hormone** (FSH), both secreted by the pituitary gland, control the development and function of the corpus luteum cells. If the egg is not fertilised, the corpus luteum ceases production of progesterone and degenerates. If the egg is fertilised, the corpus luteum continues production of progesterone until the placenta can take over this function; the corpus luteum then degenerates.

*King's Applied Anatomy of the Abdomen and Pelvis of Domestic Mammals*, First Edition. Geoff Skerritt.
© 2022 John Wiley & Sons Ltd. Published 2022 by John Wiley & Sons Ltd.
Companion website: www.wiley.com/go/skerritt/abdomen

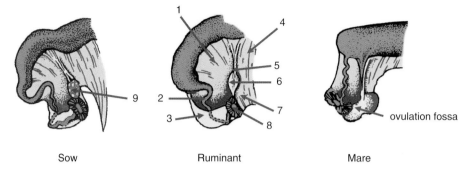

Sow           Ruminant           Mare

**Figure 13.1** The ovarian bursa – ventral views of the right ovary. 1 = mesosalpinx; 2 = uterine tube; 3 = ovarian bursa; 4 = mesometrium; 5 = proper ligament of ovary; 6 = ovary; 7 = mesovarium; 8 = infundibulum; 9 = follicles.

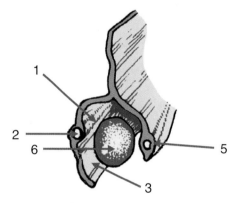

**Figure 13.2** Diagrammatic transverse section of the basic ovarian bursa. 1 = mesosalpinx; 2 = uterine tube; 3 = ovarian bursa; 4 = mesometrium; 5 = proper ligament of ovary; 6 = ovary; 7 = mesovarium; 8 = infundibulum; 9 = follicles.

## 13.2 Species Variations

### 13.2.1 Mare (Figure 13.1)

The horse's ovary is spherical in shape, except for a depression on the dorsal aspect. This is the **ovulation fossa** (Figure 13.1) and is found only in the horse. The mesothelium of the peritoneum extends over the whole surface of the ovary except at the ovulation fossa. In all the other domestic mammals, and in the human, the peritoneal epithelium of the **mesovarium** is converted, where it joins the ovary into a special low cuboidal epithelium, the so-called 'germinal epithelium'.

The ovary of the mare is very large, being the largest in the domestic mammals. A mature but sexually inactive ovary is about 6 cm in diameter. The active ovary, during oestrus, is much larger – about 9 cm in diameter. The horse's ovaries are located at the level of the third or fourth lumbar vertebrae, in the dorsal abdomen and cranioventral to the tuber coxae.

In all the other domestic animals, and in the human, the follicles are located in the cortex. In the mare they are scattered throughout the depth of the stroma. Mature follicles in the horse are very large, being up to 7 cm in diameter and containing 50–80 cc of fluid. Ovulation occurs only in the ovulation fossa; in the other domestic mammals ovulation can occur anywhere on the ovarian surface.

The corpora lutea are also very large in the horse (<5 cm), but they do not project from the surface of the ovary and are always deep within the stroma. Another feature that is peculiar to the Equidae is that at about 40 days of pregnancy a new crop of follicles appear; they may or may not ovulate but do form new (secondary) corpora lutea. Both primary and secondary corpora lutea persist until 150 days of pregnancy and then regress. Pregnancy then continues without any corpora lutea.

### 13.2.2   Cow (Figure 13.1)

The ovary of the ox is oval and flattened. It is much smaller than the ovary of the horse; it is about 3.5 cm long, 2.5 cm wide and 1.0 cm in breadth but larger when a corpus luteum is present.

The ovaries are located about halfway along the pelvic inlet, about 40 cm from the vulva and ventral to the iliac shaft. However, the position of the ovaries depends on the number of pregnancies there have been, becoming more ventral and cranial with time. When mature, the follicles are about 1 cm in diameter and project slightly from the surface of the ovary.

The corpora lutea are larger than mature follicles (2.5 cm). At 7 days the corpus luteum protrudes prominently from the surface of the ovary, enabling it to be recognised on rectal examination. If pregnancy occurs, the corpus luteum gradually sinks below the surface until it is no longer visible without cutting into the ovary. The corpus luteum of pregnancy regresses to leave a **corpus albicans** that is paler and larger than the remnant of the cyclical corpus luteum, which is reddish brown in colour and termed a **corpus rubrum**. This should not be confused with a corpus haemorrhagicum (see Section 13.1), which contains a central cavity and with a blood clot resulting from ovulation of a follicle.

In ruminants there is an intimate anatomical relationship (including actual anastomoses) between the convoluted ovarian artery and the ovarian veins, resembling the **pampiniform plexus** of the male (see Section 16.4). This arrangement facilitates the transfer of prostaglandins produced by the uterus to reach the ovary and cause termination of the corpus luteum.

### 13.2.3   Ewe (Figure 13.1)

The ovaries of the sheep are almond-shaped and 1.5–2.0 cm in length. They are located at the pelvic inlet close to the external iliac artery. As in the cow the ovaries become more cranial with successive pregnancies. In other respects the ovaries and corpora lutea are similar to those of the cow.

### 13.2.4   Sow (Figure 13.1)

In both sexually immature and mature pigs the ovary is a regular oval shape, but the surface becomes studded with either knob-like corpora lutea or with follicles that resemble a raspberry. The ovary is about 5 cm in length and is located a short distance lateroventral to the pelvic inlet. They become more ventral with successive pregnancies.

Both the follicles and the corpora luteum can be very numerous, corresponding to the size of the litter. It is not unusual for there to be as many as 24 follicles between the two ovaries. After ovulation about 18 corpora lutea may form and be associated with 12 conceptuses. The follicles and the corpora lutea both project from the surface of the ovary and are 0.5–1.0 cm in diameter.

### 13.2.5   Bitch

The shape of the immature bitch's ovary is regularly oval. When sexually active the ovary becomes lumpy with follicles and corpora lutea. In a long period of inactivity (**anoestrus**) the old corpora lutea become fibrotic, causing distortion of the ovary. The inactive ovary is 1.0–1.5 cm long in a bitch of about 15 kg. The ovaries are located ventral to the third lumbar vertebra and are quite dorsal in the abdomen, associated with short mesovaria and the straight Y-shaped **cornua** of the uterus (Figure 14.4). The ovaries are closely anchored to the last one or two ribs by the suspensory ligaments of the ovaries (see Section 3.4.3); these have to be ruptured to enable the surgeon to elevate the ovaries when carrying out an ovariectomy.

The ovarian follicles are multiple and projecting, as in the sow, but are proportionately smaller. The corpora lutea are pink in colour.

### 13.2.6   Queen

The general anatomy of the ovary is similar to that of the bitch, with a proportionate reduction in size. The mesovarium is longer in the cat than in the dog, allowing easier access to the suspensory ligament of the ovary.

## 13.3   The Ovarian Bursa (Figure 13.1)

The ovarian bursa is a pocket of peritoneum that encloses the ovary; its lumen is continuous with the peritoneal cavity via a slit-like orifice on the medial side. The **uterine tube** (**Fallopian tube** or **oviduct**) perforates the wall of the bursa and opens as the funnel-like **infundibulum** to receive the ovulated oocytes.

The degree to which the bursa encloses the ovary varies with the species. In the horse the ovary is certainly enclosed, whereas in the ruminants it is hardly enclosed at all. The pig does have a bursa, though not complete, and in the dog the ovary is tightly wrapped within the bursa. Another feature of the bursa in the bitch is that it is heavily loaded with fat, making it difficult to see the ovaries during ovariectomy. In the cat the absence of fat and the elongated **mesovarium** make surgical removal more straightforward.

## 13.4   The Uterine Tube, also called the Fallopian Tube or the Oviduct (Figure 13.2)

The **infundibulum** is the funnel-shaped ovarian end of the uterine tube; it contains fringe-like **fimbriae** that conduct the ovulated oocytes into the uterine tube. The uterine tube is about the same length in the horse, ox and pig (20–25 cm). In the dog it is very short (about 6 cm). However, tubal transit is quickest in the pig (48 hours) and slowest in the dog (4–5 days).

In the ox and pig the cornual end of the uterine tube arises from the gradually tapering uterine cornu. In the dog and cat the uterine tube arises more abruptly from the rounded end of the cornu, and in the horse it arises on a small papilla at the rounded end of the cornu.

# 14

# The Uterus, Uterine Tube, Vestibule and Vagina

## 14.1 The Uterine Cornu

The **uterus** comprises the two uterine cornu (or horns), the uterine body and the cervix. The uterus receives the fertilised ovum or ova, which become **blastocyst(s)** before implanting in the endometrium of the uterine wall. The developing embryo attaches to the uterus by a **placenta** (see Section 14.5), which allows the nutrients to pass from the maternal blood vessels to the blood of the foetus. The uterus comprises three layers. The outer layer is a serosa that is continuous with the visceral peritoneum and the mesometrium of the broad ligament. The middle layer (myometrium) consists of circular and longitudinal muscle fibres. The inner layer is the thick mucous membrane of the endometrium and includes a columnar epithelium and tubular glands.

The uterus is suspended by the **broad ligament** (Section 3.4.3), a peritoneal fold that is attached to the dorsal abdomen and the walls of the pelvis. There are three divisions of the broad ligament, according to their uterine attachments, i.e. **mesovarium, mesosalpinx** and **mesometrium**. There is usually a substantial deposit of fat in the broad ligament.

Mammalian uteri are classified according to their structure. There are four main types of uterus as follows:

**Simplex:** The entire uterus is fused into a single organ. Found in primates including human beings.

**Duplex:** There are two separate uterine bodies and cervixes but a shared vagina and vestibule. Found in marsupials, rodents and rabbits.

**Bipartite:** There are two separate uteri for most of their length but there is a shared uterine body, cervix and vagina. Found in ruminants, horses and cats.

**Bicornuate:** The upper parts of the uterus remain separate but the rest of the uterus is fused as a single organ. Found in pigs, dogs, elephants and whales.

### 14.1.1 Species variations

**Mare (Figure 14.1):** The uterine cornua are arranged in a flattened T shape, the ovarian extremities of each cornu being rounded and blunt rather than tapered. The cornua are relatively short compared with the other domestic species.

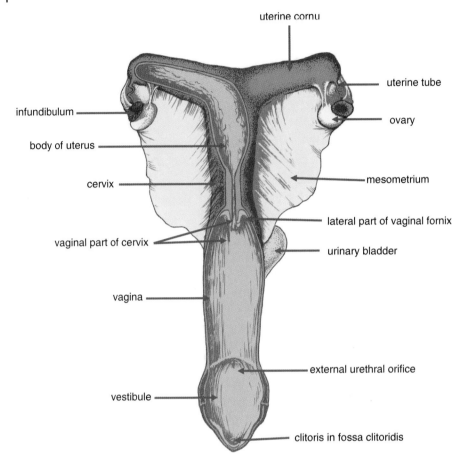

uterine cornu

uterine tube

infundibulum

ovary

body of uterus

cervix

mesometrium

lateral part of vaginal fornix

vaginal part of cervix

urinary bladder

vagina

external urethral orifice

vestibule

clitoris in fossa clitoridis

Figure 14.1 Dorsal view of the female reproductive organs of the mare. The ovaries have been rolled over so that the opening of the ovarian bursa is visible.

Since the placenta is **diffuse** (see Section 14.5), the mucous membrane is the same all over and contains many branched and coiled mucus-secreting glands. A localised region about the size and shape of a horseshoe and containing raised patches becomes apparent at about 25 days of gestation. These are the **endometrial cups**; they are about 3 cm in diameter with a central depression and disappear around halfway through pregnancy. The cells of the endometrial cups secrete equine chorionic gonadotrophin (equine luteinising hormone).

Isolated, acellular, oval objects may be present floating within the amnion or allantois. These are the **hippomanes** and occur in the ox, sheep and pig but most often in the horse. They are flattened and smooth. They are 2.5–10 cm in length and light brown in colour. Their significance is unknown, but it is suggested that they have aphrodisiac properties.

**Cow (Figure 14.2):** The uterine cornua are curled caudally so that the ovaries are close to the body of the uterus and the shaft of the ilium. The cornua gradually taper into the uterine tube. The length of the uterus is relatively long (35 cm).

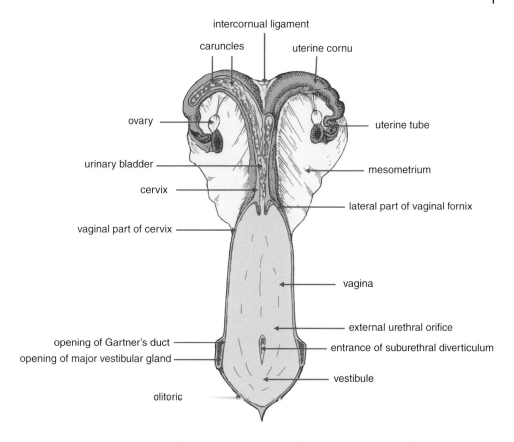

intercornual ligament

caruncles

uterine cornu

ovary

uterine tube

urinary bladder

mesometrium

cervix

vaginal part of cervix

lateral part of vaginal fornix

vagina

external urethral orifice

opening of Gartner's duct

entrance of suburethral diverticulum

opening of major vestibular gland

vestibule

clitoris

**Figure 14.2** Dorsal view the reproductive organs of the cow. The ovaries have been rolled over so that the opening of the ovarian bursa is visible.

The placenta of the cow is **cotyledonary** (see Section 14.5) and consists of about 100 **caruncles** on the endometrium that form attachments with the **foetal cotyledons**. A single unit of a caruncle and a cotyledon is called a **placentome**. In the non-pregnant state the caruncles are inconspicuous oval knobs about 1.0 cm in diameter. During pregnancy they can reach 10.0 cm in length and are attached to the uterine wall by a stalk containing their blood vessels. The removal of retained foetal membranes involves the risk of pulling off caruncles with inevitable haemorrhage. In the non-pregnant uterus the surface of the caruncles is smooth. In pregnancy the surface of the endometrium is pitted with a sponge-like network of deep crypts that accommodate the villi of the **allantochorion** (see Section 14.5).

The **intercornual ligament** (Figure 14.2) is well developed in the ox and is usually double at its cranial end; it binds the diverging cornua together.

**Ewe:** The uterine cornua of the sheep resemble those of the ox, but they are smaller. Black pigmentation of the caruncles and uterine tubes is common but not always present; a small uterus of a calf with no pigmentation resembles that of a ewe. The pregnant

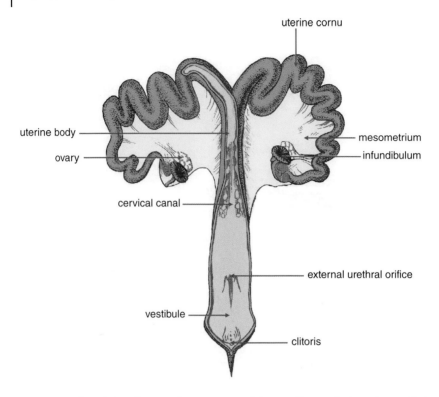

uterine cornu

uterine body

ovary

mesometrium

infundibulum

cervical canal

external urethral orifice

vestibule

clitoris

Figure 14.3 Dorsal view the reproductive organs of the sow. The ovaries have been rolled over so that the opening of the ovarian bursa is visible.

caruncles are circular with a deep depression in the centre. The intercornual ligament is single in the ewe.

**Sow (Figure 14.3):** The uterine cornua are very long in this species (<60 cm) and loosely arranged in coils. The cornua of the non-pregnant uterus resemble the thick-walled small intestine. The tip of each cornu gradually tapers into the uterine tube. The pig has a **diffuse** placenta (see Section 14.5), the surface being uniform throughout.

**Bitch (Figure 14.4):** The cornua are arranged in a Y shape and are relatively very long. Cranially each ends quite bluntly as in the horse. The endometrium includes long, relatively unbranched and straight glands. The mucous membrane is uniform in the non-pregnant uterus but the placenta is **zonary** (see Section 14.5).

**Cat:** The general features and the mucous membrane are the same as in the dog. The mesometrium often contains large quantities of fat, a feature that is useful for finding the uterine cornu when spaying a cat.

## 14.2   The Body of the Uterus (Figures 14.1–14.4)

In all the domestic mammals, except the horse, the body of the uterus is very short (ox, <6 cm; pig 5 cm; dog 2.5 cm) and of little functional importance compared with the cornua. In the horse it is much longer (almost as long as the cornua; about 20 cm) and quite capacious.

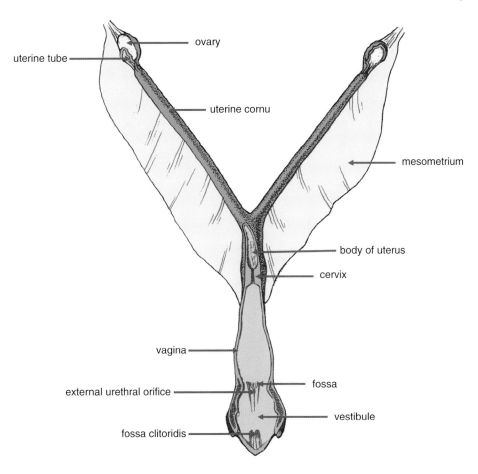

**Figure 14.4** Dorsal view the reproductive organs of the bitch.

In the cow the mesometrium is attached ventrally to the cornua and body so that the uterus can be 'picked up' on rectal examination. In the mare the mesometrium is attached dorsally, and neither the cervix nor the body can be picked up, although they can be palpated.

## 14.3  The Pregnant Uterus

### 14.3.1  Species variations

**Horse:** The foetus is equally shared between one uterine cornu and the body of the uterus. The remaining cornu is normally only slightly distended by foetal membranes. However, there can be a tendency for the foetus to extend into the other cornu. In rare cases the foetus is contained within the body and both cornua, potentially resulting in the foetus being presented transversely at birth.

As the foetus increases in size the uterus extends cranioventrally, displacing the intestines and subsiding onto the floor of the abdomen. Eventually the pregnant uterus advances as far cranially as the xiphoid cartilage and diaphragm.

**Ox and Sheep:** The foetus occupies one cornu only. The other cornu is slightly enlarged by some of the foetal membranes, which pass through the body of the uterus and into the non-gravid cornu.

As the uterus enlarges it sinks to the ventral body wall and advances along the abdominal floor. Usually it lies to the right of the rumen and enters the supraomental recess alongside the intestines; sometimes it passes ventral to the great omentum instead of entering the supraomental recess (see Section 3.2). As it grows in size the pregnant uterus displaces the rumen dorsally and to the left. Occasionally the uterus passes to the left of the rumen, displacing it to the right.

**Pig, Dog and Cat:** In all of these species there are several ovulations at each oestrus, often occurring unequally in the two ovaries. However, the foetuses are usually divided between the two cornua. This balance is achieved by migration of ova from one side to the other.

The increasing weight of the pregnant uterus causes it to sink to the abdominal floor and expand cranially towards the diaphragm.

## 14.4 Placentation

Placentation is the development of an organ that facilitates physiological exchange between the maternal and embryonic blood circulations. The organ is collectively called the placenta and comprises maternal and foetal components. The umbilical cord provides the connection between the foetus and the placenta. The cord consists of connective tissue that usually surrounds two **umbilical arteries** and two **umbilical veins** in the domestic mammals although, in humans, there is only one umbilical vein. The possession of a placenta in pregnant mammals allows development of the foetuses to an advanced stage. Marsupials also develop placentae, but the foetuses abandon intrauterine development at an early stage to continue development in the mother's pouch.

The mammalian placenta allows the transfer of nutrients and oxygen from the maternal blood to the foetal circulation. It also allows the excretory products such as uric acid, urea, creatinine and carbon dioxide to be transferred to the maternal circulation for excretion. Another valuable function of the mammalian placenta is the transfer of antibodies to the foetus.

There are four morphological types of mammalian placenta derived from the type of intimate attachment between the foetal allantochorion and the maternal endometrium:

1) **Zonary:** This type of placenta is found in dogs and cats. Other examples are bears, elephants and seals. The gross appearance of the placenta is a band encircling the middle of the foetus. Dogs and cats are usually multiparous so that the pregnant uterus appears as a series of bulges.
2) **Diffuse:** Almost all the allantochorion contributes to the placenta. Seen in pigs and horses.

3) **Cotyledonary:** Multiple 'islands' of allantochorion are present. The foetal component of each unit consists of a foetal cotyledon and a maternal caruncle, together
called a placentome. This type is seen in ruminants.
4) **Discoid:** A single disc-shaped placenta seen in primates and rodents.

### 14.4.1   The foetal membranes

The extra-embryonic or foetal membranes of the domestic mammals develop in apposition to the inner lining of the maternal uterus. They are:

1) **Yolk sac:** More correctly called the umbilical vesicle. In higher mammals it does not
contain yolk. The yolk sac develops extra-embryonically but is joined to the embryonic gut via the vitelline duct. The junction closes before birth but may still be
located as a small blind-ended vestige of the vitelline duct called **Meckel's diverticulum**, best defined in the horse.
2) **Amnion:** The amnion is a thin, tough membrane forming a fluid filled sac that surrounds the embryo except at the umbilicus. The amnion has a protective role and
combines with the outermost membrane, the chorion, to form the amniotic sac.
3) **Chorion:** This is the outermost foetal membrane. It comprises two layers, an outer
trophoblast and inner mesoderm. It develops chorionic villi early in the embryo's
development and becomes vascularised as the placenta.
4) **Allantois:** The allantois of the domestic mammals develops as a diverticulum of the
embryo's hindgut. The allantois becomes fused with the chorion and promotes rich
vascularisation. It also becomes an extension of the urinary bladder and stores
nitrogenous waste. The connection between the urinary bladder and the allantoic
sac is the **urachus**, allowing liquid waste to be passed to the allantois for storage or
voidance to the maternal blood by the placenta.

## 14.5   The Cervix Uteri (Figures 14.1–14.4)

The cervix uteri, or neck of the uterus, is the section of the reproductive tract between
the body of the uterus and vagina. In all species except the sow it projects somewhat
into the cavity of the vagina. Around this projection there is an annular space (except in
the sow) called the **vaginal fornix**. The cervix comprises a thickened firm wall of dense
fibrous tissue and both longitudinal and circular smooth muscle. Internally the cervical
canal opens into the body of the uterus via the internal **uterine os**, and into the vagina
via the external uterine os. The canal is tightly closed except during oestrus and parturition. When closed the canal is sealed with a mucus plug.
    The peritoneum is reflected from the female reproductive organs just caudal to the
cervix, making the vagina almost entirely retroperitoneal.

### 14.5.1   Species variations

**Horse:** The cervical canal is straight and about 7 cm long. It is lined by longitudinal
folds, and the vaginal part forms a rounded projection into the vagina. During copulation semen is introduced into the cervical canal or directly into the uterus. The straight

canal and the longitudinal folds enable a catheter to be passed easily in artificial insemination. The collagen of the cervix softens during pregnancy, but contraction of the smooth muscle of the cervix ensures that the canal remains closed until parturition. The cervix can actively relax in a few minutes at parturition.

**Ox:** The cervix has three or four prominent circular or spiral folds that project caudally (towards the vagina) and tend to interlock with each other. The vaginal part of the cervix is partly fused ventrally with the floor of the vagina so that the vaginal fornix is reduced ventrally but well developed dorsally. The cervical canal is longer than in the mare.

The bull ejaculates into the cranial end of the vagina. The circular folds of the cervical canal make it more difficult to pass a catheter through the canal than in the mare. During parturition the fibromuscular wall of the cervix softens abruptly, allowing the cervix to be dilated passively by the foetus during birth.

**Sheep:** The cervix of the ewe resembles that of the cow. There are five or six caudally directed circular folds. The vaginal cervix is more prominent than in the cow, consisting of irregular folds projecting further into the vagina and with a slit-like opening.

Ejaculation is into the cranial end of the vagina. Artificial insemination is not usually feasible in the ewe because of the impossibility of rectal guiding of a catheter through the cervical folds.

**Pig:** The sow's cervix is much longer than in the other species (15–20 cm). In addition to the usual longitudinal folds, there are rows of stud-like projections, each about 1.0 cm in diameter, that interlock with one another. These reduce in size until they hardly exist at either end of the cervix. There is no projection of the vaginal cervix nor a vaginal fornix.

Semen is deposited within the cervical canal, the spiral free part of the penis locking in the canal.

**Dog and Cat:** In the domestic carnivores the cervix is short and spindle-shaped. There are typical longitudinal folds. Because the cervix slopes caudoventrally, the uterine opening is dorsal and the vaginal opening is ventral; the vaginal fornix is just a small recess on the floor of the vagina.

Semen is usually ejaculated into the cervical canal. The anatomy of the cervix makes catheterisation of the uterus difficult so that semen is deposited around the vaginal cervix in artificial insemination.


## 14.6   The Vagina (Figures 14.1–14.4)

The vagina is the section of the female tract between the cervix and the vestibule. The cranial end of the vagina is enclosed by peritoneum. The peritoneal recess that lies between the vagina and rectum is the **rectoperitoneal pouch**; the corresponding recess between the vagina and the urinary bladder is the **vesicogenital pouch**. The rest of the vagina is retroperitoneal, and the vagina is within the pelvic cavity. The vaginal cervix projects into the vagina in all the domestic species except the pig; this forms the recess of the **vaginal fornix** when present.

The lining epithelium of the vagina is a stratified squamous mucous membrane that is thrown into longitudinal folds. This epithelium thickens and cornifies during proestrus and oestrus, the cornified cells being shed after oestrus.

## 14.7    The Vestibule (Figures 14.5–14.8)

The vestibule is the part of the female reproductive tract that extends from the labia of the vulva to the urethral orifice; cranially the tract continues as the vagina. When visible the hymen is a transverse membrane just cranial to the urethral orifice. The vestibule rises craniodorsally from the vulva, and among the domestic species it is longest in the pig (10 cm). The mucous vestibular glands lubricate the vestibule in copulation and parturition.

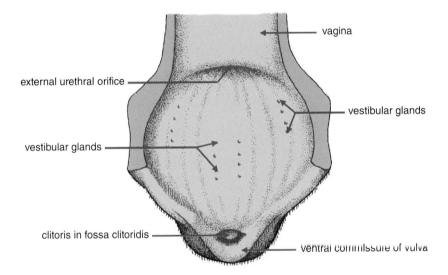

**Figure 14.5** Dorsal view the vestibule of the mare.

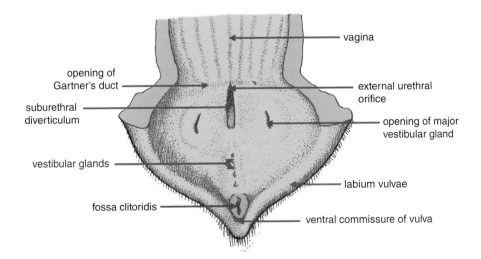

**Figure 14.6** Dorsal view the vestibule of the cow.

### 14.7.1  Species variations

**Mare (Figure 14.5):** The **external urethral** orifice is easily located. The glans clitoridis is much larger than in the other domestic mammals; it is a conspicuous, smooth, rounded body, about 1.5 cm in diameter and visible during micturition. It is located within the **fossa clitoridis**. Swabs for the diagnosis of the notifiable disease contagious equine metritis are taken from the fossa clitoridis.

The hymen is not usually visible. Two rows of vestibular glands are visible.

**Cow (Figure 14.6):** The external urethral orifice is slit-like and is located cranioventral to the large **suburethral diverticulum** in which the actual urethral opening is found. **Gartner's ducts** (remnants of the mesonephric ducts) open either side of the urethral orifice. The fossa and glans clitoridis are small and not easily located.

The vestibular glands open along a midline ventral groove. In addition, there is a single compound gland on each side termed a major vestibular gland.

**Sow (Figure 14.7):** The external urethral orifice is bounded laterally by thick folds. Gartner's glands may be present. The hymen is rarely identifiable. Two rows of vestibular glands are present.

**Bitch (Figure 14.8):** The external urethral orifice opens on a midline ridge, the urethral tubercle, and has a fossa on either side. The glans clitoridis is small and lies within a deep fossa. The fossa clitoridis may be mistaken for the **external urethral orifice** when catheterising the urethra. The vestibular glands open in two lines ventrally.

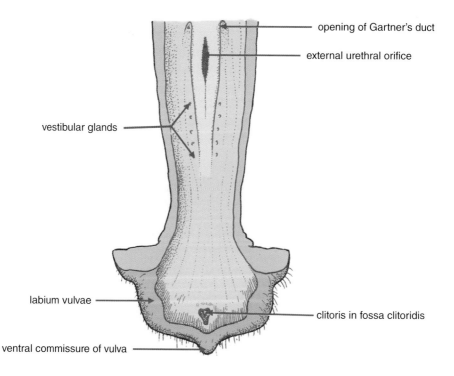

Figure 14.7  Dorsal view the vestibule of the sow.

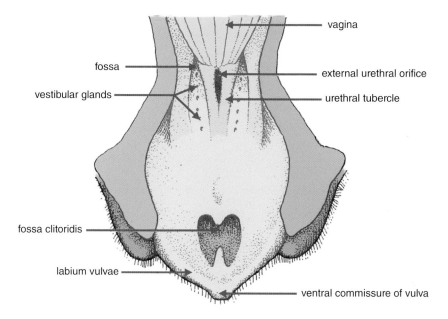

Figure 14.8 Dorsal view the vestibule of the bitch.

## 14.8 Clinical Conditions

The most significant uterine disease in the domestic mammals is **cystic endometrial hyperplasia** (CEM) in the dog. This is a common condition of entire bitches that do not become pregnant. Following oestrus, high levels of progesterone are attained, resulting in thickening of the endometrium and the development of cysts. If pregnancy does not occur, the changes in the endometrium render it vulnerable to bacterial invasion (especially by *Escherichia coli*), and large volumes of pus may result. This condition is called **pyometra**, a serious life-threatening situation. The clinical signs of pyometra are swelling and discomfort of the abdomen, usually a vaginal discharge, anorexia and excessive thirst. There is usually a high elevation of the blood white cell count. The preferred treatment is the surgical removal of the uterus and ovaries. Pyometra does occasionally occur in the cat.

In cattle the foetal membranes and placenta are expelled within 3–8 hours of parturition and certainly by 24 hours. If this does not occur the membranes are considered to be retained. Although the membranes begin to be putrid, it is now considered to be advisable not to manually remove them because of possible damage to the uterus and severe haemorrhage. Untreated cows will usually expel the membranes within 2–10 days.

# 15

# The Mammalian Penis

The male genitalia comprise the penis, testicles and accessory glands. In association are the prepuce, blood vessels and urethra.

## 15.1 The Penis

This has two functions as both the copulatory organ and the external urethra. During copulation the erect penis can enter the female vagina (intromission), allowing the ejaculation of semen into or at the entry to the cervix. The penis is normally flaccid but becomes erect prior to copulation.

To carry out its function the penis includes an extrapelvic extension of the urethra along which urine and semen may pass. It is constructed of tissue that can become engorged with blood, resulting in erection.

The penis comprises the **body** (or shaft) and the two **crura** (the root of the penis), which are each attached to an ischium on either side of the bony pelvis (os coxae). The distal portion of the penis is extrapelvic and is covered by the **prepuce**; in most species the distal extremity of the penis is expanded as the **glans penis**. The urethra is a tube lying along the midline within the penis; it conducts either semen or urine as required. The prepuce is a cutaneous sheath that covers the free part of the non-erect penis.

## 15.2 Erectile Tissue

The erectile tissue consists of two components as follows. There are marked species differences in regard to their structure and relative size.

### 15.2.1 Corpus spongiosum penis

This is a sleeve of erectile tissue that encloses the urethra from the pelvis to the distal extremity of the penis. It is expanded distally as the glans penis and near the pelvis as the **bulb** of the penis (urethral bulb).

*King's Applied Anatomy of the Abdomen and Pelvis of Domestic Mammals*, First Edition. Geoff Skerritt.
© 2022 John Wiley & Sons Ltd. Published 2022 by John Wiley & Sons Ltd.
Companion website: www.wiley.com/go/skerritt/abdomen

### 15.2.2 Corpus cavernosum penis

This erectile tissue is attached bilaterally to the left and right ischiatic tuberosities of the pelvis. It comprises a pair of fibrous cylinders that converge distally to form a single corpus cavernosum penis that lies dorsal to the urethra and extends distally to the end of the penis. This description is accurate for most species but does not apply to the dog (see Section 15.5.5).

The composition of the erectile tissue of the corpus cavernosum penis varies with the species. In man and the horse, it consists largely of smooth muscle with large cavernous spaces; this is the **musculocavernous** type of penis. The **fibroelastic** type, comprising fibrous and elastic tissue with small cavernous spaces, is found in the pig and the ruminants. During erection the release of neurotransmitters results in dilation and relaxation of the vascular components of the erectile tissue. Contraction of both the **ischiocavernosus** and **bulbospongiosus** muscles then blocks the escape of the increased blood flow, resulting in hardening of the penis, or tumescence.

During erection the musculocavernous type of penis increases greatly both in length and diameter. The fibroelastic penis undergoes straightening of the S-shaped bend in the body of the penis, the **sigmoid flexure**.

## 15.3 The Muscles of the Penis

There are three muscles that aid the function of the penis.

### 15.3.1 Retractor penis muscle

This is a narrow, elongated development of largely smooth muscle. It is connected to the internal and external sphincter muscles of the anus and also with the coccygeal muscles. The retractor penis muscle lies ventral to the body of the penis and has a loose attachment halfway along its length. The name of this muscle suggests an important function, but it is not essential for retraction of the penis into its sheath.

### 15.3.2 Ischiocavernosus muscle

This powerful paired muscle consists of striated fibres. It originates from the ischiatic arch and inserts on the **tunica albuginea** (see Section 15.5.1), a thick layer of fibrous and elastic fibres surrounding the corpus cavernosum penis, and not to be confused with the fibrous layer enclosing the seminiferous tubules of the testis. The function of this muscle is to prevent venous blood from leaving the penis during erection. In addition, its rhythmic contractions increase the pressure within the corpus cavernosum penis so that erection can be complete.

### 15.3.3 Bulbospongiosus muscle

The bulbospongiosus muscle is a thick midline, circular, striated muscle. It overlies the bulb of the penis, i.e. the caudal enlargement of the corpus spongiosum. This muscle obstructs drainage of venous blood from the corpus spongiosum and raises the pressure by rhythmic contractions. The function of this muscle is to raise the pressure within the urethra by rhythmic contractions. Such pressure pulses constrict the urethra and result in ejaculation of the semen.

## 15.4   The Blood Supply and Venous Drainage of the Penis

In all the domestic species the main supply of arterial blood to the penis is via the **internal pudendal artery**, a branch of the internal iliac artery (see Section 8.1.10 and Figure 8.2). The internal pudendal artery terminates as the artery of the penis that immediately gives rise to three branches, namely the dorsal artery of the penis, the artery of the bulb of the penis and the deep artery of the bulb.

The internal pudendal artery bends around the ischial arch and gives rise to several branches that supply the corpus spongiosum and the corpus cavernosum. The internal pudendal artery then continues as the **dorsal artery of the penis** and is located external to the tunica albuginea (see Sections 15.3.2 and 15.5.1). In most species the corpus spongiosum and the corpus cavernosum drain into the internal iliac vein via the pudendal vein (see Sections 9.1 and 9.1.3 and Figure 9.1). There are normally no vascular connections between the corpus spongiosum and the corpus cavernosum.

## 15.5   Species Variations of the Penis

### 15.5.1   Horse (Figures 15.1, 15.2a and b and 15.3)

The penis of the horse is cylindrical and slightly flattened laterally. It is about 45 cm long and 5 cm in diameter. During erection the penis doubles in length. The glans penis is the enlarged free end of the penis comprising erectile tissue that is an expanded extension of the corpus spongiosum; it caps the distal end of the corpus cavernosum penis. There are several components of the glans in this species; they are the **fossa glandis, collum glandis, corona glandis** and **urethral process**. The paired retractor penis muscle lies ventrally in the midline almost along the whole length of the body of the penis. The corpus spongiosum is covered entirely by the bulbospongiosus muscle. The trabeculae of the corpus cavernosum penis contain bundles of smooth muscle orientated longitudinally (Figure 15.2b). Sympathetic nerves maintain these in a state of tonic contraction and thereby hold the penis within the prepuce. Parasympathetic activity is responsible for erection and also inhibits the sympathetic tonic contraction.

Externally there is a strong fibroelastic capsule called the tunica albuginea (see Section 15.3.2 and Figure 15.2b). This type of penis is termed 'musculocavernous' because of the smooth muscle and the large spaces of the corpus cavernosum penis.

The urethral part of the penile body lies ventral to the corpus cavernosum penis and external to the tunica albuginea. In this species the corpus spongiosum is enclosed throughout its length by the bulbospongiosus muscle (Figure 15.2b).

There is an additional arterial supply to the penis in the horse; it is provided by the external pudendal and obturator arteries. There is a substantial drainage of venous

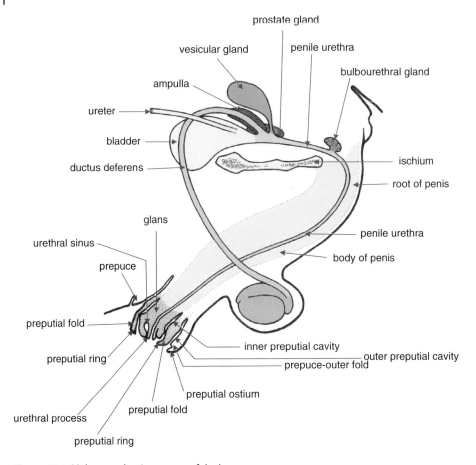

Figure 15.1 Male reproductive organs of the horse.

blood from the penis via the external pudendal vein, which passes through the inguinal canal to enter the external iliac vein. In addition, there is venous drainage via the obturator vein to the internal iliac vein.

### 15.5.2 Ox (Figures 15.4 and 15.5)

The penis of this species is virtually circular in transverse section. The diameter is smaller than that of the horse (2.5 cm) while its length is much greater (1 m.). When the penis is relaxed there is an S bend, the sigmoid flexure, which is post-scrotal in position (Figure 15.4). The tunica albuginea is reinforced by a strong non-elastic fibrous tissue layer; it encloses the corpus spongiosum as well as the corpus cavernosum. The latter is almost entirely fibrous, with only small areas of erectile tissue remaining. The body of the penis is quite firm but does contain some elastic tissue. Therefore the penis of the ox is classified as 'fibroelastic'. During erection this type of penis hardly shows any increase in diameter. The main effects of the increased blood flow are to straighten out the sigmoid flexure and to harden the glans. The sigmoid flexure returns passively to its

(a)

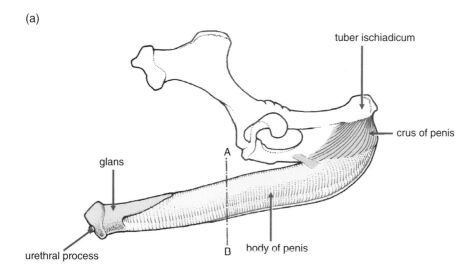

(b)

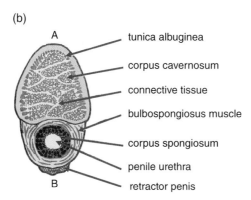

**Figure 15.2** (a) Penis of the horse. (b) Transverse section through the body of the penis of the horse at the level A-B in (a).

S shape in the non-erect penis. The retractor penis contributes little to the return of the penis to its non-erect state.

At the tip of the penis the glans penis is an enlarged helmet-like region, which, unlike that of the horse, is not a continuation of the corpus spongiosum. The urethral process is attached to the glans but does not project freely from it.

In the ox there are occasionally abnormal vascular connections that allow leakage from the corpus cavernosum into the corpus spongiosum. In this situation erection fails to occur.

### 15.5.3 Sheep (Figure 15.6)

The crura and body of the penis are similar to those of the ox. The glans penis is relatively larger than that of the ox. The **urethral process** is a worm-like extension of the

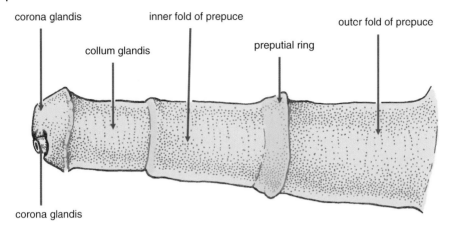

Figure 15.3 Left lateral view of the glans penis of the horse, protruded from the prepuce.

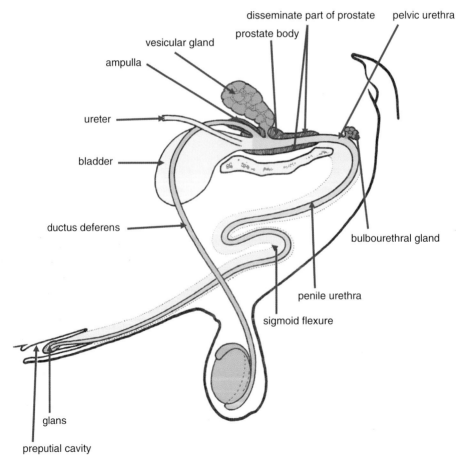

Figure 15.4 Male reproductive organs of the ox. The outline of the body of the penis is indicated by dotted lines.

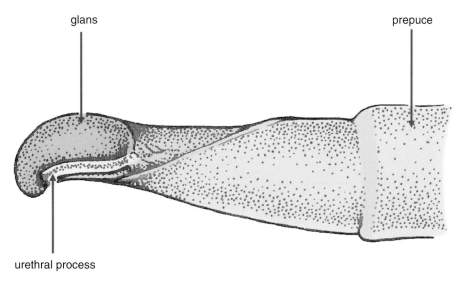

Figure 15.5 Left lateral view of the penis of the ox, protruded from the prepuce.

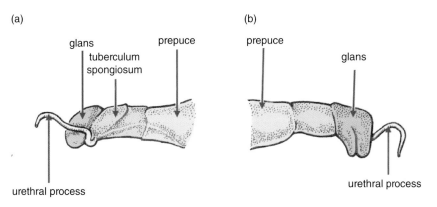

Figure 15.6 The free part of the penis of the sheep, protruded from the prepuce. (a) Left lateral view and (b) right lateral view.

urethra beyond the glans; it is about 2 cm in length. Uroliths can cause an obstruction to urethral function and require surgical removal or amputation of the process. The **tuberculum spongiosum** is an asymmetrical rounded projection of the corpus spongiosum penis on the left lateral aspect of the free part of the penis.

### 15.5.4  Pig (Figures 15.7 and 15.8)

The penis of this species is similar to that of the ox in that it is fibroelastic and comprises two crura and a body. However, the sigmoid flexure is prescrotal since the scrotum is virtually subanal in position. There is no glans penis in the pig, the free part being spirally twisted, slightly flattened and ending in a point. The urethral orifice is a slit-like

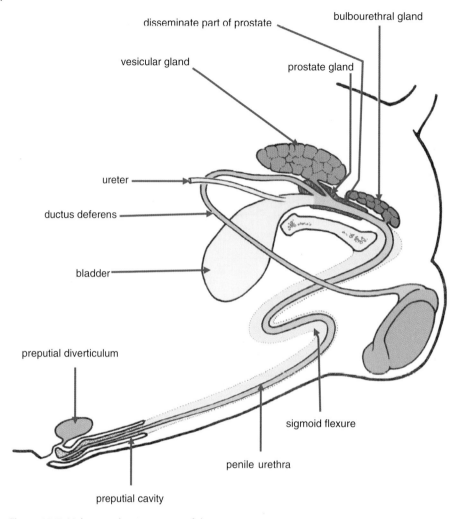

Figure 15.7  Male reproductive organs of the pig.

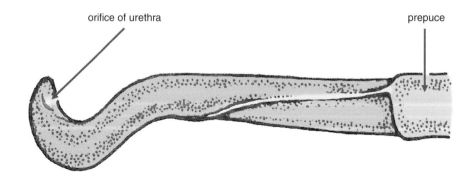

Figure 15.8  Ventral view of the free part of the penis of the pig, protruded from the prepuce.

opening near the pointed tip. There is no urethral process as in the ruminant. The pig squirts urine rather than as a continuous stream.

The boar can ejaculate up to 400 ml and take 5–10 minutes to do it.

### 15.5.5 Dog (Figures 15.9 and 15.10)

This species demonstrates several structural differences as compared with the other species.

1) Whereas there are paired crura that fuse as the body of the penis, in the caudal half of the penis the left and right corpora cavernosa penis remain separated by a midline septum.
2) The cranial part of the corpora cavernosum penis is completely ossified and has no erectile tissue; it is called the **os penis**. The urethra, enclosed in the corpus spongiosum, fits in a ventral groove in the os penis. The os penis ends just before the cranial end of the non-erect glans penis. The corpus cavernosum does not have a significant role in erection, but the erectile tissue is supplied with blood by the pudendal artery and drains via the internal pudendal vein.
3) The corpus spongiosum penis also differs from that in the other species. There are two large expansions of the corpus spongiosum: (i) the **bulbus glandis** located at the level of the caudal os penis, and (ii) the **bulb of the penis** located between the crura. It is the bulbus glandis that plays an important role during intromission.

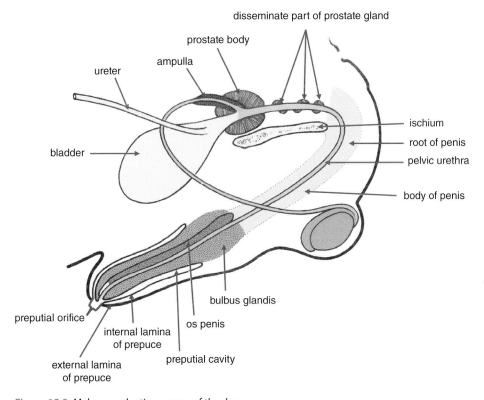

Figure 15.9 Male reproductive organs of the dog.

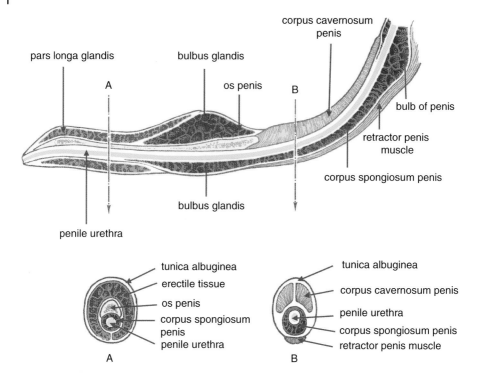

Figure 15.10 Penis of the dog with transverse sections through the glans at A and through the body of the penis at B.

The glans penis of the dog consists of the bulbus glandis and the **pars longa glandis**. The latter is the most distal (cranial) part of the corpus spongiosum, extending from the bulbus glandis to the tip of the penis. During erection the pars longa glandis increases in length.

Intromission is possible before complete erection is achieved through the stiffness of the penis conferred by the os penis. Complete erection occurs after intromission and involves enlargement of the bulbus glandis within the vestibule of the bitch. Once this is achieved it is not possible to withdraw the penis for 5–45 minutes after ejaculation.

### 15.5.6   Cat (Figure 15.11)

The penis of this species is similar to that of the dog apart from the following features.

The non-erect penis points caudally (instead of cranially as in the dog). The preputial orifice is ventral to the scrotum, which is subanal. During erection the penis pivots at its root so that the glans becomes directed cranially.

There is an os penis, but it is quite short. The glans is short and studded with small cornified barbs that serve to hold the penis firmly in the vestibule of the female.

### 15.6   The Prepuce (Figure 15.1)

This is the cutaneous sheath that covers the distal extremity of the flaccid penis. It comprises an inner and an outer lamina that are continuous with one another at the

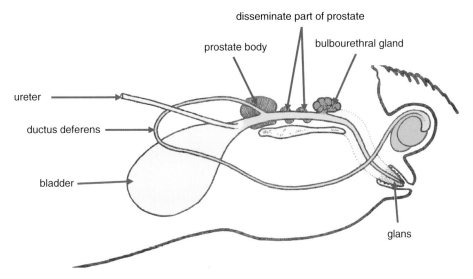

Figure 15.11  Male reproductive organs of the cat.

**preputial orifice**. The outer layer is continuous with the skin covering the body of the penis. The space between the prepuce and the body of the penis is the **preputial cavity**. When the penis is erect, the prepuce retracts to expose the glans penis and the distal part of the body of the penis.

### 15.6.1   The muscles of the prepuce

There are paired muscles attached to the prepuce both cranially and caudally. The cranial preputial muscles act as a sling for the cranial end of the prepuce and seem responsible for keeping the preputial orifice closed.

The caudal preputial muscles insert into the internal lamina of the prepuce and probably retract the prepuce. In the ox these muscles may be absent and yet the prepuce is still retractable.

### 15.6.2   The blood supply of the prepuce

The prepuce is vascularised by the dorsal artery and vein of the penis and by paired branches of the caudal superficial epigastric vessels.

### 15.6.3   Species variations of the prepuce

**Horse (Figure 15.1):** The prepuce differs from that of the other domestic mammals in that it consists of two folds, one inside the other. The inner fold is the **preputial fold** and its orifice is the **preputial ring**. The main opening is the preputial orifice. During erection both folds are stretched out to cover the shaft of the penis.

**Ruminants (Figure 15.4):** In the ox the preputial tube is long, and in the sheep it is relatively short.

**Pig (Figure 15.7):** There is a dorsal **preputial diverticulum** of the cranial part of the preputial cavity. It contains a foul-smelling liquid that has to be avoided during evisceration after slaughter. The diverticulum is rudimentary in young pigs.

**Dog and Cat (Figures 15.9 and 15.10):** There are no special features.

# 16

# The Testes

## 16.1 The Anatomy of the Testes

The paired testes, or testicles, are the male gonads or reproductive organs; they are ovoid in shape. The function of the testes is to produce **spermatozoa** (spermatogenesis) and the hormone **testosterone**. Both of these functions are controlled by hormones of the pituitary gland. There are several tissue layers covering the surface of the testes as described below. The internal tissue consists of the coiled **seminiferous tubules** and **Sertoli cells**. The latter are columnar epithelial cells that provide nutrition for the developing male gametes of the tubules. The cells of the seminiferous tubules develop through meiosis to become the male gametes; they are the site of spermatozoa development.

## 16.2 Species Variations (see Figure 16.1)

The testes of the bull and ram are approximately the same size (10–12 cm long and 250–300 g) and hang vertically in the scrotum. The stallion's testes hang almost horizontally.

## 16.3 The Scrotum

The scrotum is a sac of skin containing the testes and their outer layers. In male ruminants the scrotum is long and pendulous with a marked neck. In the stallion it is more globular with a poorly defined neck. In these animals the scrotum lies ventral to the cranial pelvis. The scrotum of the boar is almost subanal and is not well-defined, as it lies close against the caudal surface of the thighs. In the dog the scrotum is situated between the thighs and towards the anus. In the cat the scrotum is subanal.

The arterial supply of the scrotum is provided by branches of the external pudendal artery, and the nerve supply originates from the second and third lumbar (third and fourth in the dog) nerves with a small contribution from the preputial and scrotal branch on the pudendal nerve.

*King's Applied Anatomy of the Abdomen and Pelvis of Domestic Mammals*, First Edition. Geoff Skerritt.
© 2022 John Wiley & Sons Ltd. Published 2022 by John Wiley & Sons Ltd.
Companion website: www.wiley.com/go/skerritt/abdomen

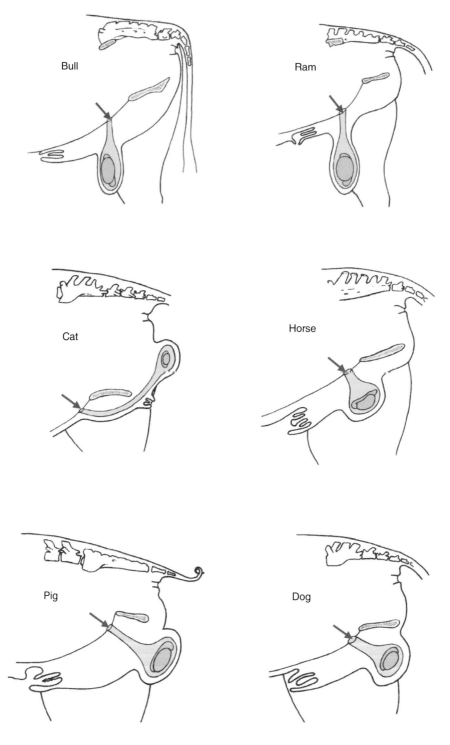

**Figure 16.1** Position of the scrotum, angle of suspension of the testis and direction of the penis in various domestic animals. The arrows point to the vaginal tunic passing through the superficial inguinal ring.

## 16.4   The Tissue Layers of the Testes and Scrotum (Figure 16.2)

1) The innermost layer, covering the seminiferous tubules, is the **tunica albuginea**. This is a tough white fibrous tissue that is continuous with the **mediastinum testis**, a cord of connective tissue lying centrally and longitudinally in the testes.

2) The next layer, lying over the tunica albuginea, is the **visceral vaginal tunic**. This fibrous layer is continuous with the visceral peritoneum through the **vaginal ring**. The vaginal tunic is essentially a diverticulum of the peritoneal cavity.

3) The parietal peritoneum is continued through the vaginal ring as the **parietal vaginal tunic**. Together with the visceral vaginal tunic it forms a flask-like sac that is reflected over the testis and epididymis distally and covering the testicular vessels and **ductus deferens** proximally. The testicular blood vessels are suspended within the cavity of the vaginal tunic by a fold of the parietal peritoneum called the **mesorchium**; it is attached to the dorsal body wall. The mesorchium is actually a wide sheet with a thickened cranial border containing the **pampiniform plexus**, the **testicular artery** and the lymphatic vessels. Medially there is a fold in the mesorchium that contains the ductus deferens. The caudal edge of the mesorchium is continuous with the parietal layer of the vaginal tunic. It is important to realise that the cavity of the vaginal tunic is continuous with the peritoneal cavity via the vaginal ring.

4) Three fascial layers derived from the muscles of the abdominal wall are next. They are the **external spermatic fascia** (external abdominal oblique muscle), the **cremasteric fascia and muscle** (internal abdominal oblique muscle) and the **internal spermatic fascia** (transverse abdominal muscle). The internal spermatic fascia is closely adherent to the outer layer of the peritoneum of the vaginal process (the vaginal tunic). The entire assembly of the cremaster muscle and fascia, the internal spermatic

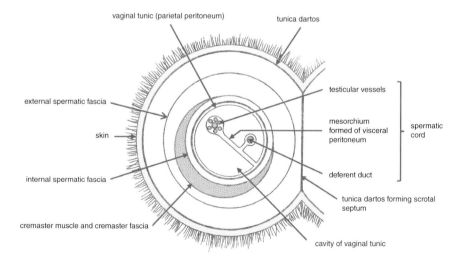

Figure 16.2   Diagrammatic cross section through the neck of the scrotum. The vaginal tunic is strongly reinforced by the closely adherent and much thicker internal spermatic fascia. In life the only potential space is the cavity of the vaginal tunic. All other layers shown in the diagram are closely apposed to their neighbours. Note that this diagram does not show a cross section of a testis.

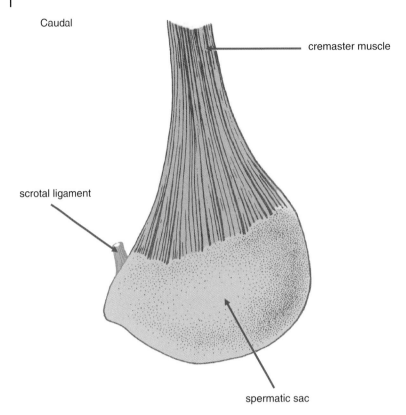

Caudal

cremaster muscle

scrotal ligament

spermatic sac

Figure 16.3 Lateral view of the right spermatic sac of the horse. The sac is hanging as it would in a standing horse in which the skin, dartos and external spermatic fascia have been dissected away during castration. The spermatic sac is a thick membrane. It consists of the vaginal tunic strongly reinforced by fusion with the thick internal spermatic fascia distally and the cremaster muscle proximally.

fascia and the vaginal tunic is called the **spermatic sac** (Figures 16.3 and 16.4). When a 'closed' castration is performed, the whole sac is dissected free of the outer layers of the scrotum. The cavity of the spermatic sac is continuous with the peritoneal cavity so that an 'open' castration gives access to the lumen of the peritoneal cavity with a risk of infection and requiring closure and control of haemorrhage with an emasculator.

5) The penultimate layer is the **tunica dartos**, comprising mainly fibroelastic tissue and smooth muscle. The dartos gives rise to the midline scrotal septum. The scrotal ligament attaches the dartos to the spermatic sac. The external spermatic fascia is loosely adherent to the dartos and is easily separated from the cremasteric fascia when performing a closed castration.

6) The outermost layer is the thin and elastic skin. In the horse there are a few hairs, whereas the scrotum of the sheep is covered with wool ventrally. Sebaceous and sweat glands are present, and there is a pigmented midline present in the horse.

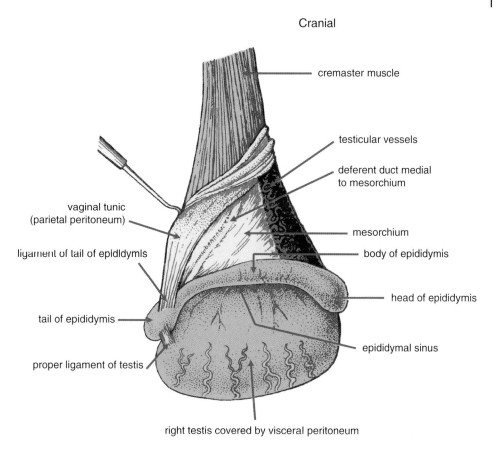

Cranial

cremaster muscle

testicular vessels

deferent duct medial
to mesorchium

vaginal tunic
(parietal peritoneum)

mesorchium

ligament of tail of epididymis

body of epididymis

head of epididymis

tail of epididymis

epididymal sinus

proper ligament of testis

right testis covered by visceral peritoneum

Figure 16.4 Lateral aspect of the contents of the right spermatic sac of the horse. The most ventral part of the spermatic sac as shown in Figure 16.3 has been incised so as to enter the lumen of the vaginal tunic.

## 16.5   The Blood Supply and Drainage of the Testes

The testicular (spermatic) artery descends in the cranial border of the spermatic cord to supply the testis; it becomes highly coiled as it reaches the testicle and is surrounded by a complex of small veins that comprise the pampiniform plexus. This intricate arrangement is called the **testicular vascular cone** and is the means by which heat exchange is enabled between arterial and venous blood. The temperature difference has been measured at 2–6°C. The testicular artery passes along the attached surface of the testis, giving rise to branches to the testis and the epididymis. It turns around the caudal pole of the testis and passes back along the convex ventral border of the testis. Its course over the testis is flexuous, and it gives off branches that ascend and descend in a tortuous fashion over the whole surface of the testis.

   The arterial supply of the scrotum is provided by branches of the external pudendal artery, and the nerve supply originates from the second and third lumbar (third and fourth in the dog) nerves with a small contribution from the preputial and scrotal branch of the pudendal nerve.

## 16.6   The Epididymis

The epididymis is a long coiled tube that both stores the spermatozoa and conducts them from the testicle to the **ductus deferens**. It is adherent to the attached border of the testis, overlapping part of the lateral surface. Macroscopically it is divided into the relatively enlarged head and tail, which are separated by the slender body.

   The head is attached to the testis by the efferent ducts of the testis and the visceral vaginal tunic. The body is only loosely separated from the visceral vaginal tunic and creates a pocket (epididymal sinus) of the vaginal tunic between the testis and the body of the epididymis. The tail of the epididymis is attached to the caudal testis by the proper ligament of the testis and to the ligament of the tail of the epididymis. Both ligaments are within folds of the visceral tunic. The tail is continued as the ductus deferens, which passes through the inguinal canal within a fold of peritoneum detached from the **mesorchium**. The cremasteric (deferent) artery and vein lie alongside the ductus deferens.

## 16.7   Species Variations (Figure 16.5)

### 16.7.1   Horse

The body is as thick as the head, and the tail projects caudally. The epididymis lies dorsally almost entirely on the testis.

### 16.7.2   Ruminant

The head of the epididymis is dorsal but is barely palpable. The body is long and slender and lies medially, between the testes alongside the ductus deferens. The tail is knob-like and projects ventral to the testis.

### 16.7.3   Pig

The head is large and projects cranially. The body is more slender than that of the horse and the tail is proportionately large and visible.

### 16.7.4   Dog

The epididymis is relatively large. The head and tail project cranially and caudally, and the body is well developed but smaller in diameter than the head and tail. The epididymis of the cat, whilst similar to that of the dog, does not project as far cranially and caudally.

## 16.8   The Descent of the Testes (Figure 16.6)

The gonads differentiate in the early embryo in the sublumbar region but, in all the domestic species, the testes migrate through the inguinal canal to the scrotum. Cryptorchidism is when one or both of the testicles fail to descend from the

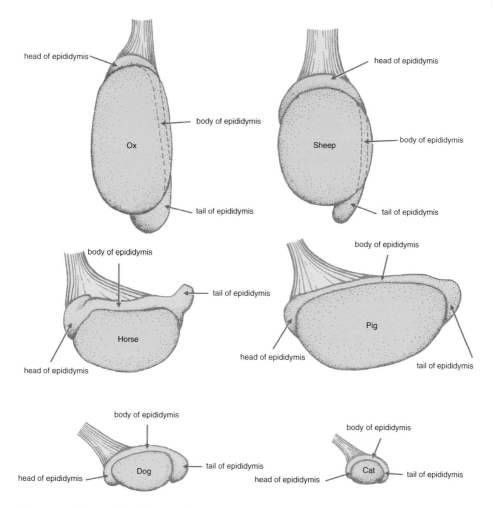

**Figure 16.5** Testis and epididymis of the domestic animals. All the drawings are of the lateral surface of the left testicle. The relative sizes are not entirely accurate. For instance the testicle of the cat is drawn much larger than it should be in relation to the large farm animals.

abdominal cavity into the scrotum. An account of the cause and the mechanism of this migration are considered here because of the incidence of cryptorchidism in the domestic animals. The process of testicular descent can be divided into four phases as follows:

1) The early stages of testicular descent result from the development of an embryonic structure, present in both sexes, called the **gubernaculum**. (See section 3.4.4) This structure is a fibrous cord (originating from mesenchyme) that, in the male, extends from the caudal pole of the testis, through the inguinal canal to attach to the distal scrotum. At this stage there is also concurrent development of the mesonephros or embryonic kidney. Despite its name and temporary function, the mesonephros does

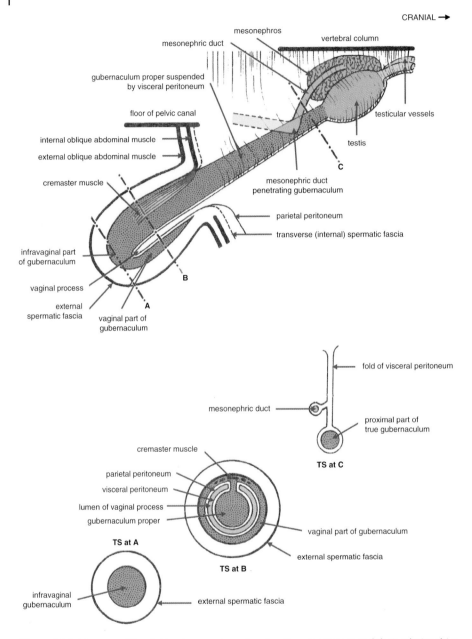

**Figure 16.6** Diagram of the right gubernaculum showing its components and their relationships shortly before the mesonephros degenrates.

not contribute to the development of the metanephros, or kidney. However, the mesonephros does give rise to the epididymis, and the mesonephric duct becomes the ductus deferens. Also at this stage of development of the gubernaculum, an evagination of the peritoneum, the vaginal process, is invaded by the gubernaculum.

2) The next phase is a transabdominal migration of the testis across the abdomen to occupy a position within the deep inguinal ring. The actual mechanism of this movement is a matter of debate. However, Gier and Marion (1969) believe that continued growth of the vaginal process distally maintains tension on an unchanging gubernaculum that, therefore, pulls the testis caudally towards the inguinal ring. By the end of this phase the mesonephros has developed into the epididymis and the ductus deferens; the cremaster muscle has developed within the vaginal part of the gubernaculum.

3) In this phase the testes pass through the inguinal ring. Formerly this descent through the inguinal ring was attributed to contraction of the gubernaculum. However, it is now accepted that this is not the case, and increase in abdominal pressure seems more significant. The testes do not become retroperitoneal during their passage into the scrotum, rather they remain encased in visceral peritoneum.

4) During this phase the gubernaculum shortens and shrinks. The infravaginal part of the gubernaculum becomes the scrotal ligament, which connects the distal part of the vaginal tunic to the scrotum. The gubernaculum proper becomes the ligament of the tail of the epididymis attaching to the distal part of the vaginal tunic. The proximal part of the gubernaculum (the part that joins the embryonic caudal pole of the gonad to the mesonephric duct) becomes the proper ligament of the testis.

## 16.9   Induction of Testicular Descent

The actual mechanism by which the descent of the testes occurs has been the subject of debate for many years and the object of much research. It is clear that there is considerable variation between species not least because of anatomical and physiological differences. Endocrine factors certainly appear to have a significant role. The requirement for the descent of the mammalian testes to an extra-abdominal location is due to the need to lower the temperature by 2–3°C of the body temperature for spermatogenesis (see Section 16.5). However, the testes of the elephant and the hyrax are intra-abdominal. Inguinal passage occurs at about 120 days of pregnancy in the ox, 80 days in the sheep and 90 days in the pig. In the horse, however, the testis is drawn to the inguinal ring, but at 100–120 days the foetal gonad starts to enlarge rapidly and is unable to pass through the inguinal canal. The gonads reach maximum size at about 210–240 days of pregnancy. The testes then undergo shrinkage until inguinal passage is possible at about 300 days, although some distortion of the testes is still necessary. By the time the foal is born the testes are normally through the inguinal canal.

# 17

# The Accessory Sex Glands

## 17.1   The Accessory Glands

This is the collective name for a number of glands associated with the male reproductive tract. The secretion of these glands is added to the semen at ejaculation, although their significance is not clear since the components of the secretion vary between species. In the immature or castrated male, the accessory glands are small.

The accessory glands comprise the single midline prostate gland, the paired vesicular glands, the single ampulla of the ductus deferens and the paired bulbourethral glands.

## 17.2   Prostate Gland

This almost spherical gland is located on the neck of the urinary bladder of male dogs. It is 1.5–2.5 cm in size, varying with the size of the dog. There are two components. The **body** of the prostate is a discrete bulbous gland lying dorsally on the neck of the bladder. The **disseminate** part of the prostate lies along the urethra. Both components have many secretory ducts. The size of the prostate varies in the domestic species, that of the dog being the relatively largest and that of the ox relatively the smallest.

### 17.2.1   Species variations

**Horse (Figure 15.1):** Only the body of the prostate is present, and in this species it is distinctly bilobed with a connecting isthmus. It is compact with multiple ducts. It lies across the neck of the bladder at the beginning of the pelvic urethra and covers the terminal sections of the deferent ducts of the vesicular glands. It comprises two lobes connected by an isthmus. The 16–20 ducts open independently on either side of the **colliculus seminalis**. The prostate is mainly retroperitoneal and can be palpated per rectum.

**Ox (Figure 15.4):** Both a body and a disseminate part are present. The body is small and slightly lobulated. The disseminate part is larger than the body but invisible

*King's Applied Anatomy of the Abdomen and Pelvis of Domestic Mammals*, First Edition. Geoff Skerritt.
© 2022 John Wiley & Sons Ltd. Published 2022 by John Wiley & Sons Ltd.
Companion website: www.wiley.com/go/skerritt/abdomen

superficially because it is covered by the urethral muscle. It opens into the pelvic urethra by a series of dorsal ducts.

**Sheep:** At a similar location to that of the ox, but only the disseminate part is present, and this is only present on the dorsal and lateral aspects of the urethra.

**Pig (Figure 15.7):** Both parts are present and resemble that of the ox, except that it is usually hidden by the large vesicular gland. The body of the prostate is small and irregularly shaped. The disseminate part lies within the wall of the pelvic urethra and discharges its secretion into the urethra through many openings.

**Dog and Cat (Figures 15.9 and 15.11):** Relatively large, comprising two hump-like lobes, and more prominent than in the other species. It surrounds the urethra and the neck of the bladder and is easily palpated per rectum in the dog owing to its large size in this species. Pathological enlargement may occur when both the rectum and the urethra may become obstructed. In these species the prostate gland produces the bulk of the seminal fluid. The two deferent ducts lie within the prostate and join the urethra within the gland. Prostatic secretion is promoted by the hypogastric nerve and up at a rate of up to 2 ml per hour.

Prostatic hyperplasia and neoplasia are common in older dogs. Inflammatory disease and prostatic abscesses occur not infrequently.

## 17.3   Vesicular Glands

This is a paired gland formerly called the seminal vesicle because it was erroneously believed to act as a reservoir for semen. Neither the dog nor the cat possess vesicular glands. The secretion is more viscous than the prostatic secretion. Histologically these glands comprise serous and muscular layers together with a mucous membrane including tubular glands. The paired openings into the urethra are located on an elevated region known as the **colliculus seminalis**.

### 17.3.1   Species variations

**Horse (Figure 15.1):** These large (15×5 cm), paired oval sacs extend cranially and dorsally on either side of the urinary bladder. The wall consists of a serous outer layer, a middle muscular layer and an inner mucous membrane containing tubular glands. The necks of the vesicular glands lie beneath the prostate gland and open together on the colliculus seminalis.

**Ox (Figure 15.4):** The paired glands are irregular-shaped lobulated masses. Though smaller than those of the pig, they are similar sized to those of the horse and take several years before reaching full size. Each gland consists of a thick-walled tube twisted and folded on itself. Compound glands are located in the wall of the tube, which opens on the colliculus seminalis.

**Pig (Figure 15.7):** The paired vesicular glands are very large and pyramidal in shape. They are lobulated and firm to the touch. There are many collecting ducts that combine to form a pair of collecting ducts that open at the colliculus seminalis. The large amount of secretion together with that of the bulbourethral gland produces the large volume of ejaculate (see Section 15.5.4).

## 17.4   Ampulla of the Ductus Deferens

The ampulla is an enlargement of the ductus deferens, although it is due to an increase in thickness of the wall rather than a dilation of the lumen of the ductus. The ampulla is absent in the pig and the cat.

**Horse (Figure 15.1):** The ampulla is relatively larger in this species (15 cm long) than in the others.

**Ox (Figure 15.4):** The ampulla is smaller than in the horse.

**Dog (Figure 15.9):** There is a poorly developed ampulla in the dog; it is largely covered by the prostate gland.

## 17.5   Bulbourethral Glands

The bulbourethral glands are paired glands that discharge their secretion into the caudal end of the urethra. They are present in all the domestic species except the dog.

**Horse (Figure 15.1):** These paired, oval glands are relatively small (5 cm). They are located beneath the urethral muscle where the pelvic urethra bends around the ischium. They are compound glands and empty into the urethra just caudal to the prostatic duct.

**Ox (Figure 15.4):** The bulbourethral glands of the ox are located at same site as in the horse, but they are smaller and have only one duct each. They are partly covered by the strong bulbospongiosus muscle. The bulbourethral glands produce a secretion that enters a diverticulum of the urethra located just caudal to the ischial arch. This secretion helps to flush the urethra prior to ejaculation.

**Pig (Figure 15.7):** These paired glands are very large in this species. They are cylindrical in shape (12 cm) and lobulated. They are compound glands with one duct each.

**Sheep:** These glands are similar to those of the ox but are relatively large. They open by a single duct in the dorsal wall of the urethra.

**Dog (Figure 15.9) and cat (Figure 15.11):** These glands are absent in the dog. They are present in cat; they are paired and pea-sized (see Figure 15.11).

## 17.6   Clinical Conditions of the Accessory Glands

Whereas the significance of the accessory glands is not clear, if they become diseased the quality of the ejaculated semen may deteriorate rapidly. In vesiculitis in the bull, white blood cells and bacteria enter the ejaculate and kill the spermatozoa. Enlargement of the prostate gland can interfere with the passage of faeces through the rectum or urine along the urethra.

## 17.7   Anal Glands

The anal sacs are located on both sides of the anus between the internal and external anal sphincter muscles. They are present only in carnivores. They are oval in shape and about 1 cm in diameter in a medium-sized dog. A short duct opens on both sides on the ventrolateral aspect of the anus. The sacs provide storage for the secretion of the coiled glands located in the wall of the sacs. The strong-smelling sebaceous secretion acts as a territory marker. Impaction of the sacs is a frequent problem requiring manual emptying.

Circumanal glands are present in a subcutaneous zone around the anus. These are also sebaceous glands but do not possess a reservoir.

# 18

# Diagnostic Imaging of the Abdomen (Figures 18.1–18.4)

Techniques available for imaging of the abdomen and the pelvis of the domestic mammals include **radiography, magnetic resonance, computed tomography and ultrasonography**. However, each technique has its application and particular indication. In general veterinary practice, it is likely that radiography will find the main use. Although all the procedures are used in the domestic species, it is in the dog and cat that they are more frequently useful with less indication for the equine abdomen because of patient size. However, diagnostic imaging is now undertaken routinely in equine practice for investigation of numerous clinical conditions including colic and weight loss. In this species it is also used for certain interventional procedures such as ultrasound-guided liver biopsy and surgical procedures such as **laparoscopic cryptorchidectomy** or **ovariectomy**. Abdominal radiography is useful in equine patients for identifying sand impactions of the large colon.

## 18.1 Radiographic Anatomy

Owing to the large number of tissues all of much the same density, there is a lack of radiological contrast between the organs of the abdomen. Air in the lungs promotes a contrast effect and greater definition in thoracic radiographs. However, the presence of fat in the abdomen provides better contrast in older or obese animals, thereby emphasising the outline of the kidneys, spleen, liver and the urinary bladder, for example. Other contrasting materials are gas and radiopaque substances within the lumen of the intestines. Large masses within the intestine may hide other organs and may necessitate emptying of the alimentary tract before radiographic study.

Since movement of the animal may cause blurring of the radiograph, sedation or anaesthesia may be necessary. Correct positioning of the abdominal organs is only obtained with the animal standing, particularly when lateral views are required. However, the usual positioning will be in lateral, sternal or dorsal recumbency.

The poor contrast between abdominal tissues may make it difficult to define a specific organ clearly. In these circumstances it may be necessary to administer a contrast medium. This is a radiopaque agent such as **barium sulphate** or a water-soluble **iodine**

*King's Applied Anatomy of the Abdomen and Pelvis of Domestic Mammals*, First Edition. Geoff Skerritt.
© 2022 John Wiley & Sons Ltd. Published 2022 by John Wiley & Sons Ltd.
Companion website: www.wiley.com/go/skerritt/abdomen

preparation. Barium is given by mouth as a colloidal suspension and is used to investigate the alimentary tract. The iodine compounds are given intravenously and are used especially to identify vascular lesions and for excretion **urography**.

Whereas in small animals good radiography will demonstrate the liver, spleen, kidneys, urinary bladder, stomach and intestines, other organs, e.g. pancreas, uterus, ovaries and lymph nodes, will not be visible unless they are grossly abnormal.

## 18.2   Specific Organs

### 18.2.1   The stomach

The dark area of the stomach represents the gas-filled area of the fundus and is situated to the left of the midline at the level of the last two ribs. The distended stomach extends caudally to the ribs and can occupy almost a third of the abdominal cavity when distended. Often the stomach has a figure-of-eight shape on lateral radiographs, indicating a state of contraction (Figure 18.2). When the stomach is not distended it is largely overlain by the liver (Figures 18.1 and 18.2).

**Oral barium** is often administered to aid the diagnosis of tumours, diaphragmatic hernias or radio-transparent **foreign bodies** such as plastic toys or fur balls in cats. The radiograph should be obtained no longer than 3 minutes after administration of the barium when the stomach is being investigated. (See Section 18.2.4 for speed of transit of barium in the intestines.)

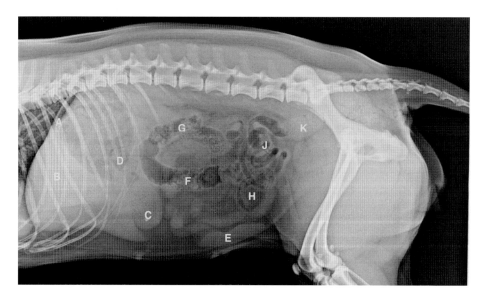

Figure 18.1 Lateral radiograph of the abdomen of a dog. A = diaphragm; B = liver; C = stomach; D = stomach; E = spleen; F = descending colon; G = ascending colon; H = urinary bladder; J = jejunoileum; K = rectum.

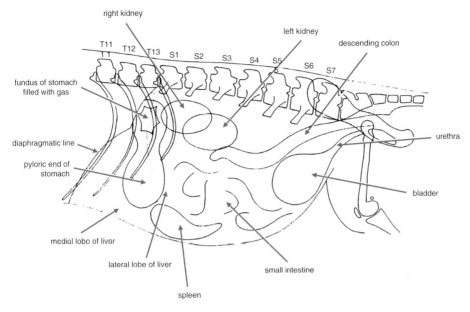

**Figure 18.2** Diagram of lateral radiograph of the abdomen of the dog in the standing position. Rarely do all of the organs show as clearly as this. Alteration of the exposure values and times improves the visualisation of the different structures.

### 18.2.2 The spleen

The spleen does vary in position depending on the fullness of the stomach. It looks conspicuously dense compared with adjacent structures due to its high content of blood. The size of the spleen can vary markedly between normal individuals and can be considerably enlarged as a result of barbiturate anaesthesia.

### 18.2.3 The liver

The liver is easily recognised as an area of relative density, although its precise outline is readily determined. Its cranial boundary coincides fairly closely with the concave diaphragmatic line. The borders of the lobes tend to merge with the stomach and the spleen.

**Cholecystography** is a radiological procedure involving the administration of an iodine compound that is administered intravenously or orally and is preferentially excreted by the liver. The result is outlining of the gall bladder and the bile, hepatic and cystic ducts radiographically. Portal venography is a contrast technique used to facilitate the radiographic appearance of portosystemic shunts (see Section 7.7).

### 18.2.4 The intestines

The large intestine is often clearly visible radiographically due to the presence within its lumen of gas, ingesta or faecal matter showing as areas of varying radiotransparency or opacity. The small intestine is not so easily distinguished, but its presence is suggested by an area of mottled opacity and the occasional gas bubble.

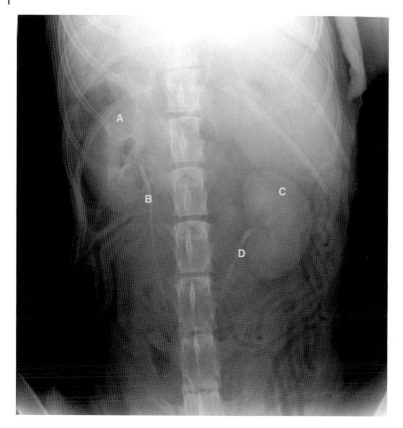

**Figure 18.3** Ventrodorsal radiograph of the abdomen of a dog. A water-soluble contrast medium has been given intravenously to show the kidneys and ureters. A = right kidney; B = right ureter; C = left kidney; D = left ureter.

Oral barium is used to show the position, and often the cause of obstructions, of the small and large intestines. It is also used for detecting tumours and the displacement of the alimentary tract.

The region of the intestine containing barium, as seen on the radiograph, depends on the time between administration and exposure. Some barium is seen in the duodenum after only 5 minutes, and the whole of the small intestine is visible after 30 minutes. The ascending and descending colon is filled by 90 minutes, and the barium remains within the descending colon and the rectum until defaecation. A better technique for the visualisation of the large intestine is the administration of a barium enema since immediate and post-evacuation radiographs give an accurate clinical study; the caecum is particularly well seen by this procedure.

### 18.2.5   The kidneys

To obtain optimum radiography of the kidneys, the alimentary tract should first be emptied as completely as possible. The kidneys are well demonstrated on a lateral film, although there is some overlap (see Figure 18.2). In ventrodorsal radiographs there is

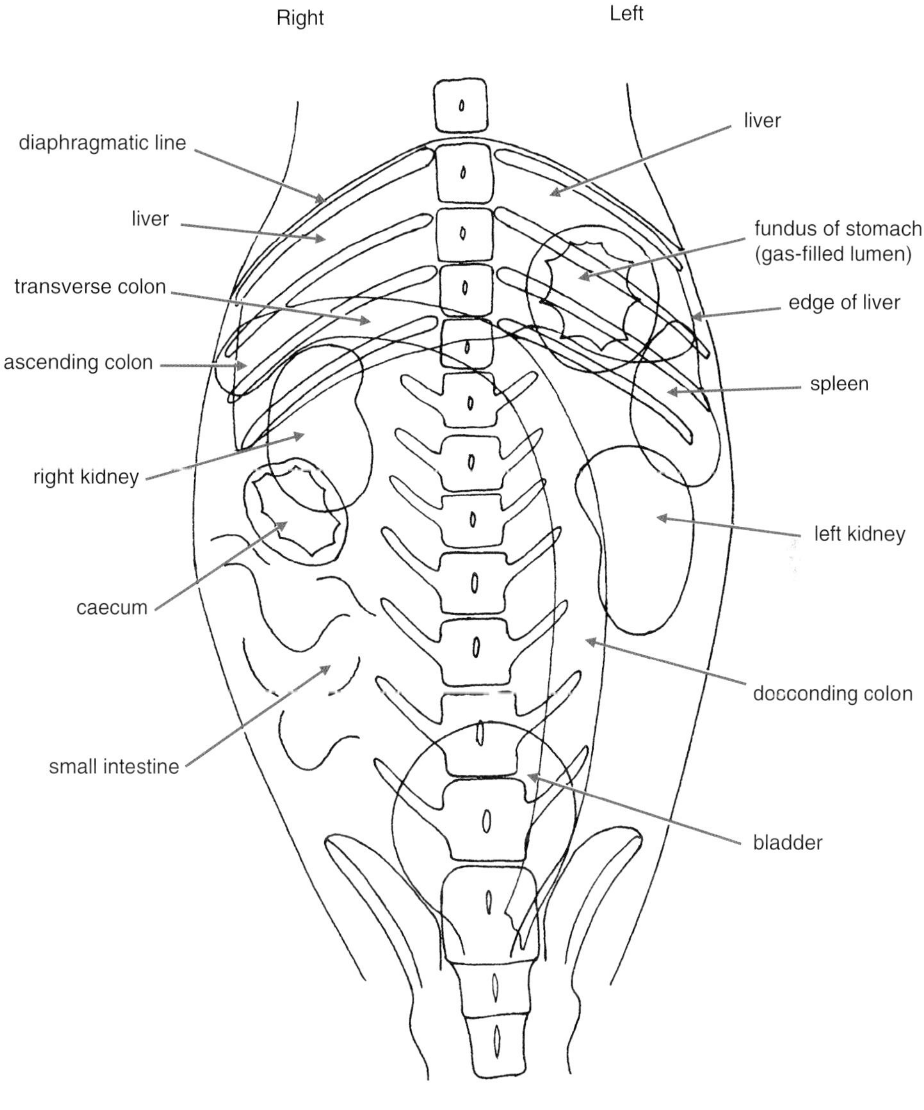

Right                                         Left

diaphragmatic line

liver

liver

transverse colon

fundus of stomach
(gas-filled lumen)

edge of liver

ascending colon

spleen

right kidney

left kidney

caecum

descending colon

small intestine

bladder

Figure 18.4 Diagram of ventrodorsal radiograph of the abdomen of the dog.

some obscuring superimposition by the liver (right), spleen (left), caecum (right) and the lumbar muscles. Variations in size, tumours and, sometimes, **renal calculi** may be identified without the use of contrast media.

Although there is little application in veterinary practice, the kidneys are well demonstrated by **pyelography** (urography). The technique involves the intravenous administration of an organic water-soluble iodide, preferably under anaesthesia. Apart from radiopacity of the kidneys, the renal end of ureters is rendered radiopaque.

The introduction of air into the peritoneal cavity does improve the external outline of the kidneys, but the patient does need to be in ventral recumbency.

### 18.2.6 Urinary bladder

The bladder is clearly visible in both lateral and ventrodorsal views, providing the bladder contains an appreciable amount of urine since it is difficult to see when empty.

Clinically radiography of the bladder is carried out most frequently for the purpose of detecting cystic **calculi**. However, **urate stones**, common in the Dalmatian, are not adequately radiopaque. **Pneumocystography**, a radiographic study following the introduction of air into the bladder via a urethral catheter, is a useful technique for detecting calculi.

Aqueous organic iodides may be introduced into the bladder by urinary catheter for the investigation of an obstruction or neoplasia.

### 18.2.7 Urethra and prostate gland

The urethra is not easily seen on plain radiographs, although its position is indicated by the os penis in male dogs. The main reason for its radiographic study is to demonstrate the presence of calculi, which are usually radiopaque. The prostate gland is not seen on radiographs unless it is markedly enlarged and it has dropped forward over the pelvic brim. In this position it must be distinguished from the urinary bladder.

## 18.3 Magnetic Resonance Imaging (MRI)

MRI scanning is a fairly recent development in veterinary practice, and it continues to make advances as the techniques are refined and applied. It is tempting to consider that MRI will render radiography out-dated, but this is a mistake as the techniques are

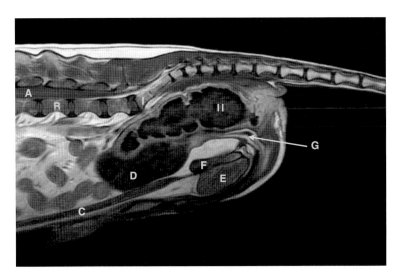

Figure 18.5 Lateral MRI scan of the pelvis of a dog. A = spinal cord; B = 5th lumbar vertebra; C = penile urethra; D = urinary bladder; E = gracilis muscle; F = pelvic symphysis; G = urethra (male); H = rectum; I = sacrum.

complementary. Even computed tomography (CT), which is closely related to radiography, will not supersede radiography in the near future.

MRI scanning requires that the production of the images takes time and that the patient must remain quite immobile whilst the scanner builds the picture, taking 5–15 minutes. Of course, radiography takes a picture like a camera and the image is then developed without involvement of the patient. Heavy sedation or anaesthesia is required as it takes the scanner 5–30 minutes to construct the image.

The MRI scanner uses a **strong magnetic field** and **radio waves** to construct an image. The magnetic field is either from a permanent magnet or a superconducting electromagnet. The former is less expensive to buy and maintain but is not as powerful in the quality of results. It is not within the scope of this book to explain how the MRI scanner produces images (see the bibliography). However, it should be pointed out that permanent magnet systems operate at a low field strength, typically around 0.25 Tesla, whereas superconducting magnets, as used in medical and veterinary diagnosis, have a field strength of 0.5–1.5 Tesla (and even 3.0 T). Basically it is the relaxation of the excited hydrogen atoms in water and fat that changes the radio signal that is being induced. It is the recovery and direction of the spinning hydrogen atoms that results in T1 and T2 relaxation, the basis of the two main types of MR image. In **T1 images** water has a low (dark) signal and fat has a high (bright) signal: in **T2 images** water has a high (bright) signal and fat also has a high (bright) signal. Since the abdomen has high concentrations of both water and fat, it is not surprising that this region gives excellent opportunities for imaging.

MRI scanning is particularly helpful for locating and assessing neoplasia and foreign bodies (Figures 18.6 and 18.7). Sometimes it is helpful to administer a contrast agent with a T1 weighted sequence so that, for example, an abnormally vascular organ or tissue will have a bright image. **Gadolinium** is a contrast agent that is used in MRI scanning of veterinary patients, although it is not licensed for veterinary use. Figures 18.5–18.7 show examples of MRI scans of the abdomen and pelvis of canine patients.

## 18.4   Computed Tomography

This is a technique that uses multiple radiographic images obtained in different planes. The images are then subjected to computer analysis to produce a series of slices through the body. The result is a very clear and detailed image in 3D. The technique is particularly useful for examination of hard tissues. For comparison of CT with MRI it has to be admitted that the soft tissues of the abdomen and pelvis are better examined with MRI, but CT is less expensive.

## 18.5   Ultrasonography

Ultrasonography for veterinary diagnosis was first employed in the late 1960s. The technique had already been used for examination of slaughter animal tissues. The first clinical application began with pregnancy diagnoses in sheep and then dogs.

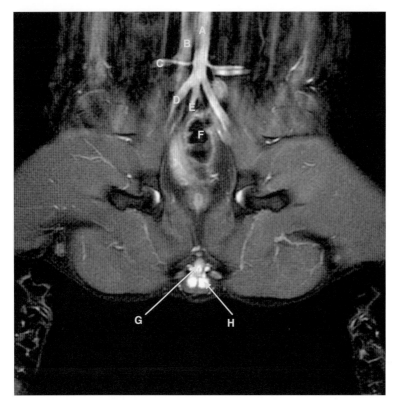

Figure 18.6 Dorsal MRI (T2W) of the pelvis of a dog. A = aorta; B = caudal vena cava; C = right deep circumflex iliac artery; D = right external iliac artery; E = right internal iliac artery; F = rectum; G = urethra; H = bulb of urethra.

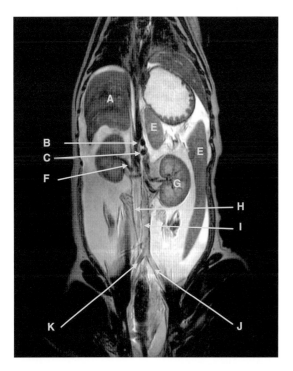

Figure 18.7 Dorsal MRI scan (T2W) of the abdomen of a dog. A = liver; B = coeliac artery; C = cranial mesenteric artery; D = stomach; E = spleen; F = renal artery; G = left kidney; H = vena cava; I = aorta; J = left external iliac artery; K = right external iliac artery.

Currently the technique is used mainly in farm animals, although there are applications in ophthalmology and pregnancy diagnosis in small animals. In recent years ultrasonography of the abdomen has almost become part of the routine diagnostic procedure.

The sound frequency employed in ultrasonography is higher than the range of human hearing. Dogs and cats can perceive ultrasound well in excess of human ability, although they do not show any disturbance at the frequencies used clinically.

The ultrasound transducer converts electrical energy to ultrasound and a computer develops images that are displayed on a computer screen. The high-frequency sound is inaudible to human ears and apparently causes no disturbance to animals. The sound waves promote echoes that bounce back from the targets, giving information on the size, shape and consistency of the soft tissues and organs. Ultrasonography is particularly useful for examinations of the abdomen from which a picture of the organs or the pregnant uterus can be prepared by the computer.

## 18.6   Diagnostic Imaging in Equine Patients

**Ultrasonography**, performed transrectally, is utilised routinely for assessment of a mare's reproductive tract, to diagnose pregnancy and to stage the oestrus cycle in mares. Small portable ultrasound machines facilitate this use in ambulatory practice, while larger more powerful machines are used for transcutaneous abdominal ultrasound. Thorough assessment of the abdomen requires low-frequency (3–5 MHz) ultrasound transducers that can scan up to depths of 20–25 cm. Numerous abdominal ultrasound protocols have been published detailing effective abdominal screening for horses with abdominal pain (colic), and abdominal ultrasound is considered routine in equine hospitals for assessment of horses with colic. Ultrasound has high diagnostic specificity and sensitivity for the identification of horses with strangulating intestinal lesions (colon volvulus and small intestinal strangulation), nephrosplenic entrapment (Figure 10.1) of the large colon, gastric impactions, displacement of the large colon and diaphragmatic hernia. Ultrasound can also detect peritoneal effusions and is commonly used in the investigation of the genitourinary systems. Ultrasound is also utilised to identify the location of retained abdominal testis and is performed routinely in horses with weight loss and/or diarrhoea. Due to the fundamental principles of ultrasound, it has limited capacity in the presence of gas-filled viscus, and imaging deep to the gas is impossible.

**Gastroscopy** in adults is performed with a 3m flexible video endoscope and is indicated in horses with suspected oesophageal and gastric disease. The procedure is performed in standing, often lightly sedated horses following at least 12 hours of fasting to ensure that the stomach is empty. Gastric ulcers are the most commonly reported gastric disease in horses and are found in the squamous portion of the stomach near the **margo plicatus** (Figure 4.1) or in the glandular portion of the stomach around the pylorus. Gastroscopy is also useful for diagnosing and monitoring response to treatment of gastric impaction and in younger horses with gastric outflow obstruction. Bot fly larvae (*Gastrophilus*) are infrequently encountered attached to the squamous portion of the stomach but are considered incidental.

**Laparoscopy** (Figures 18.8–18.10) is performed in adult horses in the standing position to access the dorsal parts of the abdomen and, under general anaesthesia, to access

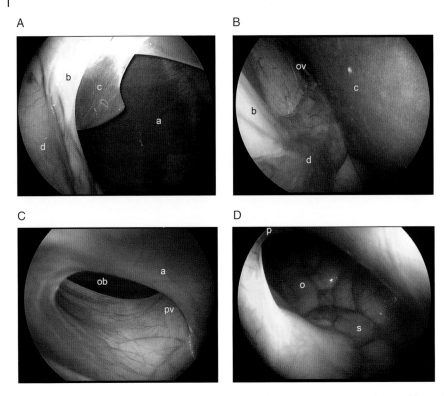

Figure 18.8 Laparoscopic examination of the epiploic foramen. Images were obtained from the right side of the abdomen. (A) The right lobe (label a) and caudate lobe (label c) of the liver lie cranial to the duodenum (label d) suspended by the hepatoduodenal ligament (label b). (B) The laparoscope is advanced between the caudate lobe (label c) of the liver and the hepatoduodenal ligament (label b) to visualise the omental vestibule (ov). (C) The laparoscope is advanced into the omental vestibule where the omental bursa (ob) is seen beyond the epiploic foramen. The portal vein (pv) lies in a ventral position at this location and is covered by serosa. (D) The laparoscope is placed through the epiploic foramen to the left side of the abdomen where the lesser curvature of the stomach (s) and omentum (o) are visible. The edge of the pancreas within the hepatopancreatic fold (p) can just be seen dorsally.

the ventral parts. Laparoscopy is performed with rigid 10 mm wide forward or forward-oblique (30°) endoscope placed through an 11 mm diameter cannula positioned in the paralumbar fossa or the 17th intercostal space. Typically, the abdomen is distended slightly with medical grade $CO_2$ to improve visualisation (pneumoperitoneum). Horses undergoing laparoscopy under general anaesthesia are often positioned in the **Trendelenburg position** (dorsal recumbency with the head down) or reverse-Trendelenburg position (head up) if greater access is required to the caudal or cranial abdomen, respectively. The main indications for laparoscopy in adult horses are **ovariectomy** of diseased ovaries (granulosa cell tumour or haemorrhaging follicles) and **cryptorchidectomy**. Closure of the epiploic foramen with mesh implants is performed in horses with previous history of epiploic foramen entrapment (see Section 3.2 and Figure 3.1). Closure of the **nephrosplenic space** is undertaken in horses at risk of nephrosplenic entrapment of the colon by suturing the spleen to the nephrosplenic

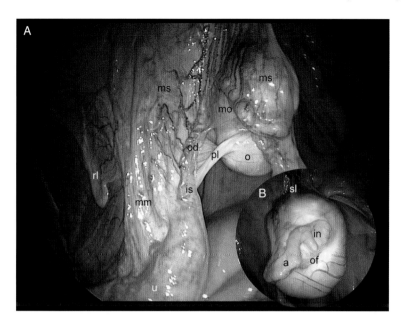

**Figure 18.9** (A) Laparoscopic view of the right ovary and cranial aspect of the right uterine horn of a mare. The laparoscope has been inserted through the right flank. (B) The inset is an image of the medial aspect of the right ovary. The ovary (o) is supported from the dorsal body wall by the suspensory ligament (sl) and mesovarium (mo) and is attached to the cranial aspect of the uterine horn by the proper ligament (pl). The uterus (u) is suspended to the dorsal body wall by the broad ligament/mesometrium (mm) and connected to the lateral body wall by the round ligament (rl). The ovulation fossa (ov) is visible on the medial side of the ovary (o) adjacent to the infundibulum (in) of the oviduct (od). The infundibulum continues as the ampulla (a) of the oviduct (od) as it wraps around the caudal aspect of the ovary (o). The oviduct continues as a convoluted tube supported by the mesosalpinx before widening at the isthmus (is) where the oviduct joins the cranial uterine horn.

ligament, and the inguinal canal of stallions can be partially closed by a variety of laparoscopically guided methods. Other less common indications for laparoscopy in adult horses include **uteropexy** (fixation of a displaced uterus), or **imbrication of the broad ligament** (surgical overlapping of the ligament) of the uterus in mares with a pendulous uterus and treatment of obstructed oviducts with prostaglandin.

With the advent of larger-bore CT scanners, imaging of the caudal abdomen and pelvis is possible in the horse, but this technique has not been investigated for this purpose to date. It is probable that abdominal CT scanning in horses will be reported in the future.

## 18.7    Diagnostic Imaging in Farm Animals

Farm animal abdominal imaging is typically reserved for investigation of urinary and gastrointestinal disease in small ruminants and pigs, although usage of ultrasound for examination of the adult bovine abdomen is increasing. Abdominal ultrasound in calves is also very useful for identification of **umbilical remnant infection**. Ultrasonography

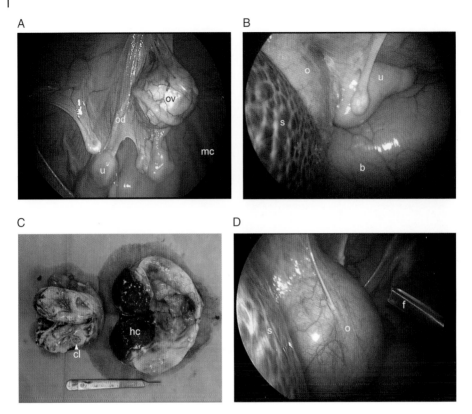

Figure 18.10 Laparoscopic images obtained via flank approach in a standing, sedated mare (A), (B), (D), and a photograph of the sectioned ovaries following laparoscopically guided ovariectomy (C). The mare had behavioural difficulties attributable to a painful left ovary. (A) The right ovary (o), oviduct (od) and uterus (u) are clearly identifiable in the right caudal part of the abdomen. The mesocolon (mc) divides the left and right caudal abdominal compartments. (B) The partially visible left ovary (o) is enlarged and lying medial to the spleen (s). The left uterine (u) horn runs caudally over the full urinary bladder (label b). (C) Both ovaries were removed and are shown following sagittal sectioning. The left ovary contains a large haemorrhagic cyst (hc), and a corpus luteum (cl) is present in the right ovary. (D) The same view as in (B) but the ovary (o) has been manipulated to lie lateral to the spleen (s) by means of an atraumatic grasping forceps (f).

and to a lesser extent abdominal and pelvic radiography are utilised to confirm diagnosis and to assess the response to treatment of obstructive **urolithiasis** in goats and occasionally sheep.

**Laparoscopic ovariectomy** is routinely performed in pet pigs and has several advantages over traditional open ovariectomy including lower morbidity and mortality. **Laparoscopic artificial insemination** is the process whereby frozen semen is inseminated deeply into the uterine horn under laparoscopic guidance. This advanced technique is undertaken by peripatetic specialists in intensive sheep-breeding outfits where synchronisation of oestrus in the ewes permits insemination of multiple ewes on the same day.

## 18.8   Laparoscopy in Dogs and Cats

Laparoscopic surgery ('**keyhole surgery**') in dogs and cats has become more available as veterinarians develop skills in the technique. There are undoubted advantages of laparoscopy not least because of the small incisions and the in situ visibility of the abdominal organs. **Ovariectomy** is certainly the most frequent application of laparoscopy in dogs and cats, but there is a disadvantage of leaving the uterus in place since uterine infections or neoplasia can still occur. However, post-operative pain is minimal, there is faster recovery time and healing is quicker.

Further applications of the technique are also being practised, for example:

1) Biopsies of the liver, kidneys and intestines
2) Exploratory surgery of the abdomen
3) Cryptorchidectomy to remove a retained testicle
4) Removal of urinary calculi
5) Arthroscopy to examine joints, e.g. for ruptured ligaments.

# Appendix

## Questionnaire

This is a multiple choice true/false questionnaire. Each question is arranged as four statements, but one of the four is false in each question. Every one of the questions can be answered from the information given in the text. The answers are given at the end.

1  **A**  All dogs have 13 pairs of ribs.
   **B**  Horses have 18 pairs of ribs.
   **C**  Pigs have 12–16 pairs of ribs.
   **D**  Sheep have 12 pairs of ribs.

2  **A**  The aorta passes between the crura of the diaphragm.
   **B**  The vagus nerves do not pass between the crura of the diaphragm.
   **C**  The caudal vena cava does not pass between the crura of the diaphragm.
   **D**  The thoracic duct does not pass between the crura of the diaphragm.

3  **A**  The rectus abdominis muscle inserts with the prepubic tendon.
   **B**  The cremaster muscle is an extension of the internal abdominal oblique muscle.
   **C**  In the dog the sheath of the rectus abdominal muscle is dorsal to the rectus abdominis.
   **D**  The transverse abdominal muscle inserts in the linea alba.

4  **A**  Intestine may herniate through the inguinal canal.
   **B**  Intestine may herniate through the umbilical ring.
   **C**  The lungs may enter the abdomen in a diaphragmatic hernia.
   **D**  Perineal hernias may occur in the dog.

5  **A**  All mammals digest cellulose by bacterial fermentation.
   **B**  Particulate matter may be removed from the gut by phagocytosis.
   **C**  The gut contents are moved through the intestine by peristalsis.
   **D**  Mucus is produced in the intestines to lubricate the passage of food.

*King's Applied Anatomy of the Abdomen and Pelvis of Domestic Mammals*, First Edition. Geoff Skerritt.
© 2022 John Wiley & Sons Ltd. Published 2022 by John Wiley & Sons Ltd.
Companion website: www.wiley.com/go/skerritt/abdomen

6  **A**  The stomach of the dog is covered by visceral peritoneum.
   **B**  The ventral sac of the rumen is within the greater omentum.
   **C**  The ovaries are covered by visceral peritoneum.
   **D**  The epiploic foramen is the only entry to the omental bursa.

7  **A**  The falciform ligament is developed from ventral mesogastrium.
   **B**  The lesser omentum is developed from ventral mesogastrium.
   **C**  The round ligament is a remnant of the umbilical vein.
   **D**  The urachus is a remnant of the amnion.

8  **A**  The greater omentum is a site for fat deposition.
   **B**  The greater omentum does not isolate foci of infection.
   **C**  The greater omentum is an insulating layer.
   **D**  The greater omentum can be used to protect surgical wounds.

9  **A**  The broad ligaments attach the ovaries to the body wall.
   **B**  The mesosalpinx is attached to the uterine tube.
   **C**  The round ligament of the uterus is the homologue of the gubernaculum.
   **D**  The proper ligament attaches the ovary to the last rib.

10  **A**  The proximal part of the stomach is developed from the oesophagus.
   **B**  The cardia of the stomach is present only in mammals.
   **C**  The fundic region of the stomach contains tubular glands.
   **D**  Cells in the pyloric region of the stomach secrete hydrochloric acid.

11  **A**  Horses are able to vomit easily.
   **B**  Ruminants chew the cud.
   **C**  The pig's stomach possesses a diverticulum of the fundus.
   **D**  Bloat is an accumulation of gas in the ruminant stomach.

12  **A**  Gastric dilatation is a frequent problem in large breed dogs.
   **B**  Gastric torsion can cause sudden death in pigs.
   **C**  Vagus indigestion occurs in ruminants.
   **D**  Shorthair cats commonly suffer from stomach hairballs.

13  **A**  Peyer's patches contain lymphocytes.
   **B**  The myenteric plexus consists of autonomic neurons.
   **C**  Brunner's glands are not found in the domestic mammals.
   **D**  The pancreatic ducts convey bile to the duodenum.

14  **A**  Johne's disease in ruminants is caused by a mycobacterium.
   **B**  Canine parvovirus can cause intestinal and cardiac disease in dogs.
   **C**  The small intestine of the ox is located on the left side.
   **D**  Intussusception is telescoping of the small intestine.

15   **A**  The appendix is an appendage of the caecum in domestic animals.
    **B**  The horse digests its herbivorous diet in the large intestine.
    **C**  There are four divisions of the large (ascending) colon in the horse.
    **D**  The ascending colon of the pig is mainly on the left.

16   **A**  There are four liver lobes in mammals.
    **B**  The gall bladder is located next to the caudate lobe in all mammals.
    **C**  The bile duct and blood vessels access the liver at the hilus.
    **D**  The cystic duct drains bile from the liver.

17   **A**  Insulin is secreted by the pancreatic islets.
    **B**  The exocrine secretion of the pancreas contains digestive enzymes.
    **C**  Ruminants have only one pancreatic duct.
    **D**  Pancreatic gamma cells produce insulin.

18   **A**  Portosystemic shunts are abnormal blood bypasses of the liver.
    **B**  Hepatitis is a viral disease in dogs.
    **C**  Liver fluke is a parasitic disease of herbivores.
    **D**  Diabetes insipidus is caused by inadequate production of insulin.

19   **A**  The dorsal aorta provides the major arterial supply to the abdomen.
    **B**  The coeliac artery provides the main blood supply to the spleen.
    **C**  Branches of the cranial mesenteric artery supply blood to the kidneys.
    **D**  The caudal mesenteric artery gives rise to the left colic artery.

20   **A**  The right azygos vein is functional in the horse.
    **B**  The portal system conveys blood to the liver.
    **C**  The caudal vena cava is the main drainage from the abdomen to the heart.
    **D**  The caudal vena cava passes through the diaphragm at the aortic hiatus.

21   **A**  Lacteals are lymphatic capillaries in the small intestines.
    **B**  The cisterna chyli is a dilation of the thoracic duct.
    **C**  The dog's spleen stores 10% of the total number of red blood cells.
    **D**  The red pulp of the spleen stores blood components.

22   **A**  Feline leukaemia can affect all carnivores.
    **B**  Lymphosarcoma is a common malignant disease of dogs and cats.
    **C**  Splenomegaly may be neoplastic or inflammatory.
    **D**  The spleen of the horse can release red blood cells in response to exercise.

23   **A**  Sympathetic motor neurons are found in the lateral horn of the spinal cord.
    **B**  The great splanchnic nerve contains sympathetic axons.
    **C**  Prevertebral ganglia are found near the coeliac artery.
    **D**  Postganglionic parasympathetic endings release adrenaline.

24  **A** The anal sphincter is innervated by the pudendal nerve.
    **B** The vagus nerve contains parasympathetic nerves.
    **C** The adrenal medulla secretes adrenaline.
    **D** The hypogastric nerve innervates the stomach.

25  **A** Renal corpuscles include glomeruli.
    **B** The loops of Henle are located in the adrenal medulla.
    **C** Gross lobation is a feature of the cow's kidney.
    **D** The kidneys are covered in visceral peritoneum.

26  **A** The canine kidneys filter up to 300 litres of blood daily.
    **B** The left kidney of the cow is on the right of the midline.
    **C** A simple columnar epithelium lines the urinary bladder.
    **D** The chromaffin cells of the adrenal medulla produce adrenaline.

27  **A** The corpus luteum of mammals produces mainly oestradiol.
    **B** Follicle-stimulating hormone is produced by the pituitary gland.
    **C** Bleeding at ovulation is from a corpus haemorrhagicum.
    **D** The follicles of the mare are located in the ovarian stroma.

28  **A** The ovarian bursa of the bitch usually contains much fat.
    **B** The mammalian uterus is suspended by the broad ligament.
    **C** The uterus of the pig is duplex.
    **D** Endometrial cups are found in the mare's placenta.

29  **A** A placentome consists of a foetal cotyledon and a maternal placentome.
    **B** The bitch has a zonary placenta.
    **C** The allantois stores the embryo's nitrogenous waste.
    **D** The mammalian placenta is unable to transfer antibodies to the foetus.

30  **A** The vestibule extends from the vulva to the urethral orifice.
    **B** Artificial insemination is possible in all ruminants
    **C** In the sow the vaginal cervix does not project into the vagina.
    **D** The cervix of the mare can be relaxed in minutes at parturition.

31  **A** The boar has a musculocavernous penis.
    **B** The retractor penis muscle consists mostly of smooth muscle.
    **C** The bulbospongiosis muscle is mainly responsible for ejaculation.
    **D** The corpus spongiosum and corpus cavernosum have vascular connections.

32  **A** In the horse the tunica albuginea surrounds the penile urethra.
    **B** In the horse parasympathetic activity is responsible for ejaculation.
    **C** In the horse sympathetic activity is responsible for retracting the prepuce.
    **D** The prepuce of the horse has two folds.

33   **A**  The urethral process of the ox projects from the glans.
      **B**  The sigmoid flexure of the ox straightens out during erection.
      **C**  The bulbus glandis of the dog maintains intromission within the vestibule.
      **D**  Cornified barbs on the cat's penis hold it firmly in the vestibule.

34   **A**  The function of the testes is to produce spermatozoa and progesterone.
      **B**  The mesorchium is a fold of parietal peritoneum.
      **C**  The spermatic sac consists of internal spermatic fascia and the vaginal tunic.
      **D**  The scrotum of the ram is covered in wool.

35   **A**  The testicular vascular cone controls the blood temperature of the testes.
      **B**  Spermatozoa are stored in the epididymis.
      **C**  The testicles of ruminants are held vertically.
      **D**  Descent of the testes is attributed to contraction of the gubernaculum.

36   **A**  The prostate gland consists of a body and a disseminate part.
      **B**  The dog and cat both possess vesicular glands.
      **C**  A large volume of secretion is produced by the vesicular glands of the pig.
      **D**  The ram has a pair of bulbourethral glands.

37   **A**  The spleen is clearly visible on a radiograph of a dog's abdomen.
      **B**  The ovaries are seen clearly on a radiograph of a cat's abdomen.
      **C**  The presence of gas in the intestines enhances a radiograph.
      **D**  Bone is seen as a distinctive pale shadow radiographically.

38   **A**  Oral barium sulphate enhances the abdominal viscera radiographically.
      **B**  Intravenous iodine compounds enhance the urinary tract radiographically.
      **C**  Urate bladder stones are seen clearly on radiographic examination.
      **D**  In pneumocystography air is used as a contrast agent in the urinary bladder.

39   **A**  Laparoscopic ovariectomy is not possible in the pig.
      **B**  Ultrasound is useful in the diagnosis of urolithiasis in the goat.
      **C**  Ultrasonography can be used to identify umbilical remnant infection.
      **D**  Pyometra can still occur in the bitch after laparoscopic ovariectomy.

40   **A**  Transrectal ultrasonography can be used to determine oestrus in the mare.
      **B**  Ultrasonography can be used to diagnose diaphragmatic hernia in the horse.
      **C**  Radiography can be used to detect the presence of sand in the large colon of the horse.
      **D**  Laparoscopic ovariectomy is not possible in the mare as the ovaries cannot be visualised.

## Answers to Questionnaire

| | | | |
|---|---|---|---|
| 1 D | 2 D | 3 C | 4 C |
| 5 A | 6 C | 7 D | 8 B |
| 9 D | 10 A | 11 A | 12 D |
| 13 D | 14 C | 15 A | 16 B |
| 17 D | 18 D | 19 C | 20 D |
| 21 C | 22 A | 23 D | 24 D |
| 25 D | 26 C | 27 A | 28 C |
| 29 D | 30 B | 31 A | 32 A |
| 33 A | 34 A | 35 D | 36 B |
| 37 B | 38 C | 39 A | 40 D |

# Bibliography

Akers, M.R., and Denbow, D.M. (2013) *Anatomy and Physiology of Domestic Animals* (2nd edn). Wiley Blackwell, Ames, Iowa.

Al-Sobayil, F.A., and Ahmed, A.F. (2007) Surgical treatment for different forms of hernias in sheep and goats. *J. Vet. Sci*, **8**(2), 185–191.

Ashdown, R.R. (1963) The anatomy of the inguinal canal in the domestic animals. *Vet. Rec.* **75**, 1345–1351.

Bates, R.O., and Straw, B. (2008) Hernias in growing pigs. *Michigan State University Pork Quarterly* **13**.

Bergin, W.C., Gier, H.T., Marion, G.B., and Coffman, J.R. (1970) A developmental concept of equine cryptorchidism 1. *Biol. Repro.* **3**, 88–92.

Bergin, W.C., Gier, H.T., Marion, G.B. et al. (1970) A developmental concept of equine cryptorchidism. *Biol. Reprod.* **3**, 82–92.

Bexfield, N., and Lee. K. (2014) *BSAVA Guide to Procedures in Small Animal Practice.* BSAVA, Gloucester.

Bojrab, M.J., Waldron, D.R., and Toombs, J.P. (2014) *Current Techniques in Small Animal Surgery* (5th edn). Teton NewMedia, Jackson, Wyoming.

Boyer, T., and Lindor, K. (2016) *Zakim and Boyer's Hepatology*. Elsevier, Amsterdam.

Brown, S.A. (2013) *Renal Dysfunction in Small Animals*. MSD Veterinary Manual, https://www.merckvetmanual.com/urinary-system/noninfectious-diseases-of-the-urinary-system-in-small-animals/renal-dysfunction-in-small-animals.

Burger, J.W.A., van t' Riet, M., and Jeekel, J. (2002) Abdominal incisions: techniques and postoperative complications. *Scand. J. Surg.*, **91**, 315–321.

Constantinescu, G.M. (2001) *Guide to Regional Ruminant Anatomy Based on the Dissection of the Goat*. Iowa State University Press, Ames, Iowa.

Constantinescu, G.M. (2002) *Clinical Anatomy for Small Animal Practitioners*. Iowa State University Press, Ames, Iowa.

Davidson, M., Else, R., and Lumsden, J. (1998) *Manual of Small Animal Clinical Pathology*. BSAVA, Cheltenham.

de Lahunta, A., and Glass, E. (2009) *Veterinary Neuroanatomy and Clinical Neurology* (3rd edn). Saunders, Philadelphia, Pennsylvania.

Dyce, K.M., Sack, W.O., and Wensing, C.J.G. (1987) *Textbook of Veterinary Anatomy*. Saunders, Philadelphia, Pennsylvania.

Elliott, I., and Skerritt, G.C. (2010) *Handbook of Small Animal MRI*. Wiley Blackwell, Oxford.

*King's Applied Anatomy of the Abdomen and Pelvis of Domestic Mammals*, First Edition. Geoff Skerritt.
© 2022 John Wiley & Sons Ltd. Published 2022 by John Wiley & Sons Ltd.
Companion website: www.wiley.com/go/skerritt/abdomen

Evans, H.E., and de Lahunta, A. (2012) *Miller's Anatomy of the Dog* (4th edn). Saunders, Philadelphia, Pennsylvania.

Fossum, T.W. (2018) *Small Animal Surgery* (5th edn). Mosby, Philadelphia, Pennsylvania.

Frandson, R.D., Wilke, W.D., and Fails, A.D. (2003) *Anatomy and Physiology of Farm Animals* (6th edn). Lippincott, Williams and Wilkins, Ambler, Pennsylvania.

Fubini, S.L., and Ducharma, N.G. (2016) *Farm Animal Surgery* (2nd edn). Elsevier/ Saunders, Philadelphia, Pennsylvania.

Getty, R. (1975) Sisson and Grossman's *The Anatomy of the Domestic Animals* (5th edn). Saunders, Philadelphia, Pennsylvania.

Gier, H.T., and Marion, G.B. (1969) Development of the mammalian testis and genital ducts. *Biol. Repro. Suppl.* **1**, 1–22.

Hafez, E.S.E., and Hafez, B. (2013) *Reproduction in Farm Animals* (7th edn). Wiley Blackwell, Ames, Iowa.

Hall. E.J., Simpson, J.W., and Williams, D.A. (2018) *Manual of Canine and Feline Gastroenterology* (2nd edn), 190–202. BSAVA, Gloucester.

Hendrickson, D.A., and Baird, A.N. (2013) Turner and McIlraith's *Techniques in Large Animal* Surgery (6th edn). Elsevier/Mosby, Philadelphia, Pennsylvania.

Mizeres, N. J. (1955) The anatomy of the autonomic nervous system in the dog. *Am. J. Anat.* **96**, 285–318.

Nautrup, C.P., Tobias, R., and Cartee, R.E. (2000) *An Atlas and Textbook of Diagnostic Ultrasonography of the Dog and Cat.* Manson Publishing Ltd., London.

Neal, P.A., and Edwards, G.B. (1968) Vagus indigestion in cattle. *Vet. Rec.* **82**, 396–402.

International Committee of Gross Anatomical Nomenclature. (2003) *Nomina Anatomica Veterinaria* (5th edn). World Association of Veterinary Anatomists, Knoxville, Tennessee.

Nyland, T.G., and Mattoon, J.S. (2002) *Small Animal Diagnostic Ultrasound* (2nd edn). Saunders, Philadelphia, Pennsylvania.

Pasquini, C., Spurgeon, T., and Pasquini, S. (1995) *Anatomy of Domestic Animals* (8th edn). SUDZ Publishing, Pilot Point, Texas.

Platt, S., and Olby, N. (2013) *Manual of Canine and Feline Neurology* (4th edn). BSAVA, Gloucester.

Rebhun, W.C. (1980) *Vagus indigestion in cattle. JAVMA* **176**, 506–510.

Richter, K.P. (2001) Laparoscopy in dogs and cats. *Vet. Clin. N. Am. Small Anim. Pract.* **31** (4), 707–727.

Sack, W.O. (1982) *Essentials of Pig Anatomy.* Veterinary Textbooks, Ithaca, New York.

Sanyal, A.J., Lindor, K.D., Boyer,T.D. and Terrault, N.A. (2018) Zakim and Boyer's Hepatology: A Textbook of Liver Disease (7th edn). Elsevier, Philadelphia.

Skerritt, G.C. (2018) *Applied Anatomy of the Central Nervous System of Domestic Mammals.* (2nd edn). Wiley Blackwell, Oxford.

Smallwood, J.E. (1992) *A Guided Tour of Veterinary Anatomy.* Saunders, Philadelphia, Pennsylvania.

Villiers, E., and Blackwood, L. (2012) *Manual of Canine and Feline Clinical Pathology* (2nd edn). BSAVA, Gloucester.

Weber, R.F. (1979) The bovine mammary gland: structure and function. *JAVMA* **170**, 1133–1136.

Wensing, C.J.G. (1968) Testicular descent in some domestic mammals, I. Anatomical aspect of testicular descent. *Koninski. Ned. Akad. Wetensch. Proc. Ser. C* **71**, 423–434.

Wensing, C.J.G. (1973) Testicular descent in some domestic mammals, II The nature of the gubernacular change during the process of testicular descent in the pig. *Koninski. Ned. Akad. Wetensch. Proc. Ser. C* **76**, 190–202.

# Index

*King's Applied Anatomy of the Abdomen and Pelvis of Domestic Mammals*, First Edition. Geoff Skerritt.
© 2022 John Wiley & Sons Ltd. Published 2022 by John Wiley & Sons Ltd.
Companion website: www.wiley.com/go/skerritt/abdomen